THE SECRET OF INDIAN HEALTH

a concept and opinion

DR. P.G. RAO

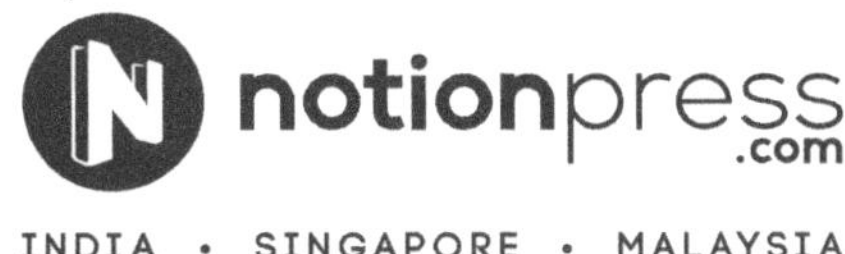

notionpress.com

INDIA · SINGAPORE · MALAYSIA

ISBN 979-8-89415-013-0

Health, a concept and opinion

Edited by
Pothukutchi Sabita Priyamvada nee Sripada

Contents

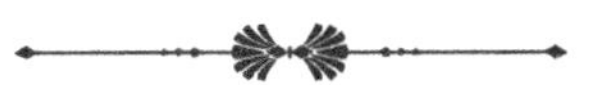

In loving memory of my late Uncle
Dr. Potukuchi Ramachandra Rao

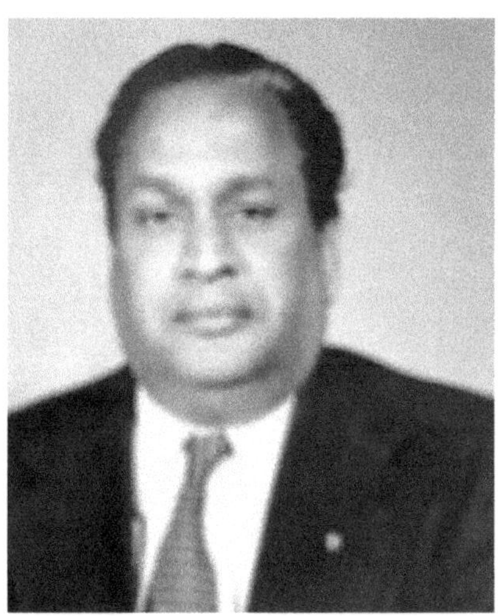

Foreword

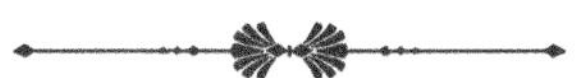

In crafting this book, "Health: Concept and Opinion," I draw profound inspiration from two extraordinary women who have profoundly shaped my understanding of holistic wellness: my late grandmother, P. Subbamma, and aunt, Potukuchi Vardhani Rao. Their mastery of simple remedies using spices and vegetables to address common health issues left a lasting impression on me. As their knowledge passed down through generations, it profoundly influenced my perspective on health and wellness.

A significant influence in my life has been my late uncle, Dr. Potukuchi Ramachandra Rao, DSc, FRIC, London. As a UNESCO expert and Professor, he served as my mentor, coach, and father figure. His guidance and wisdom have played a pivotal role in shaping me into the person I am today. I have spent a significant portion of my life with him, learning invaluable lessons that continue to guide me.

This book embodies my quest to bridge the wisdom of age-old home remedies with contemporary scientific knowledge. Through its pages, I aim to provide practical insights and actionable advice, empowering individuals to embrace natural approaches to health and wellness.

Coming into the subject, the Indian living and thinking have a blend of health, wealth, and auto-discipline. Here food, water, and health are part of systematic planning using festivals as the foundation. The traditional Indian approach to health emphasizes the use of medicinal herbs, temple worship, and a holistic view of well-being.

The ancient Indian medical system, epitomized by texts like the Sushruta Samhita and Charak Samhita, emphasized not just the absence of disease but also a healthy mind and spirit. While modern medicine has made significant strides, we must acknowledge the roots of our traditional healing practices and their relevance in today's world.

As we navigate the complexities of modern healthcare, it becomes evident that the integration of traditional wisdom with modern advancements holds immense promise. Observations on practices like long walks, fasting, and the use of natural elements such as cow dung and urine offer intriguing insights into age-old remedies that continue to hold relevance.

Furthermore, reflections on fiscal discipline, mathematical principles, and the significance of environmental factors like Vaastu underscore the interconnectedness of various aspects of life with health and wellness.

Observation I: Long walk: Adi-Shankara was the first person to walk long distances by foot. The sacred fire for Yagna or hawan is generated by him using friction of two wooden attachments- made of Ficus specie called raavi and Prosophis spicigera, called jammi! Thus, Adi-Shankara implemented an adoptable model for living- hundreds of years back.

In old days, even Mahatma Gandhi used to carry two friction stones to generate fire and once, he ordered his grand-daughter to go back to that village to get his stones back and she angrily went and brought them & threw towards her grandpa-this was a real story narrated by Mahatma's grand-daughter at SRH School, Tuni – where I was a student @ 1961-66 then.

Observation II: A sudden Crisis:

Example1: the former Prime Minister Morarji Desai survived a plane crash (in 1980's), wherein he walked five kilometres to reach a police station to introduce himself as the Prime Minister of India.

In another example,- In 1970's, a lady who survived a Boeing plane crash narrated her experience (old Reader's digest) which was horrifying as she had no access to food or medicine. She had reached the nearby village to inform the public of her survival. Thus, a regular walking habit rescued the above persons.

Observation III: Fasting: Mahatma Gandhi used to fast as a weapon in every protest. Even now, day time fasting methods are practiced for better health by several groups like Ayyapan or Hanuman or Bhavani etc., groups. Even now, people of Islamic origin adopt day-time fast during Ramzan.

Observation IV: health in (Sanskrit) sloka: In another sloka, "Dharma – artha – Kama – moksha –…. Nam – Arogyam – moolamuttamam"- means keeping good health is the best. Salvation comes through hard work & meditation-provided one survives.

Thus, the prime importance to be given in life, is health only. The English quotation- 'health is wealth'- is not different. At another place, "Satayur – vajra – dehaya – sarvasampat – karayacha – sarva – arista – vinas Aya- nimbakamdala- bhakshanam"- Take leaves of neem throughout the year, live hundred years- disease free with strong body- is the meaning of the sloka.

This was followed by Mahatma Gandhi throughout his life and he was always disease free. Swami Yogananda (when he visited mahatma Gandhi) was surprised to see Gandhi's way of consumption of Azadirachta indica or neem leaves. It means the olden methods were still prevalent then!

Why that health system collapsed? It had partially yielded to the attractive modern medicine. The very first attack by British is occupation of vacant lands, which eliminated herbs.

Observation V: The place of worship: The best way one can be clean is living like the idols-- on a regular basis and herbal farms still exist. Here ayurveda is associated with the priest as he recognizes the plant- leaves and flowers- for regular worship. In my opinion, a temple is an aesthetic place for making of some herbal drugs by hand.

The temples also provide employment to sculptors, priests, transporters, flower vendors, & even temple employees. Further, temples used to serve as a sterile place for drying, making powders, or even hand-made goli (I purchased – hand made, Tibetan medicines in Dharamshala, HP, India). In general, the priest can suggest a good herb in recovery!

Observation VI: Urine therapy: The late Prime minister of India, Morarji Desai admitted drinking of his own urine every day- a few ml. He once said that even his brother was treated in a similar way. Here, even epileptic/and insane patients are advised to drink few ml of donkey urine every day.

Adding a step further, some urines are used both externally and internally; here elephant urine – used as a wormicide, leucoderma cure; camel urine- bitter, cure asthma, cough, piles; horse urine-bitter, cure leukoderma; sheep urine – bitter and cooling; cow urine – bitter, cures leucoderma, destroy worms; buffalo urine – reduces piles, swellings, dropsy, it is alkaline and purgative; ass urine –used for epilepsy & insanity; Now also cow urine is used and panca-gavya is a vital medicine. But such urines are subject to at least seven step purifications- which critics are not aware.

Observation VII: Cow dung therapy: In another example, a person suffering from fever is asked to hold a bolus of fresh cow dung and the mantra chant begins. Technically speaking, how can mantra cure? Though, the mantra contributes some mental solace, the bolus does the rest. Thus, the bolus of cow dung is kept in the hands of the sick or diseased and mantra is uttered. Here, mantra is the time needed for bolus to act.

The patient is suggested to change to fresh cow dung during the chant. Thus, for about 108 times mantra is uttered with a chanting time of about two hours. It is enough for the digestive & excretory enzymes of fresh cow dung to enter the body. Then, the person's digestive ability improves and accumulated poisons fast digested & he even purges after the treatment. The fever gets eliminated, making the patient healthy in a couple of days.

It is common during my childhood days wherein my maternal grand- father (mother's father) used to order at home for bringing fresh cow dung for painting the mud walls of home or even to make the dried cow dung biscuits as garlands. Every child is asked to prepare separate a small garland of 108 pieces of cow dung biscuits for Lohri (bhogi) festival – means his hands are sunken in it at least for 3-4 hours- once in a year. This gives immunity to fight many diseases. These dried cow dung biscuits are offered as a garland into the fire to worship Sun, plus the ash serve as an excellent tooth powder. I used it for tooth cleaning for years.

Note: If cow dung cakes are made by machine, where is the therapy?

Observation VIII: Immunity: The final aspect is the neglected immunity, which needs to be gained. For me, the suggestion of Vemana's scribes appealed me. Here Yogi- Vemana wrote a hundred poems in Telugu. According to him, "Gangi.Govu...Paalu... Garete... Dinanu....chalu…" – means a cup milk of good age-old cow is enough. This was written several centuries ago- is worth mention. Why? Probably that small amount of milk can develop immunity mechanisms in the body.

Jenner's vaccine for small pox is a novel example. He is successful because the Indian cow breed is at least several generations of isolated animal strains.

The hybrid cows- what Yogi Vemana described as donkeys- can yield more milk, but can't produce antibody or vaccine (lack of immunity)!

Observation IX: Skin thickness: When I was awarded a gold medal by Hari-om Trust of Gujarat Ayurvedic University (GAU) Jamnagar (for the theory on bioavailability), I visited that place and attended conference. In that conference, one author suggested a direct correlation between the thicknesses of the layers of human skin to the width of the grain consumed by him (Vriha-in Sanskrit sloka).

Observation X: Vaastu is another dimension to look into our environment as Vaastu decides the shape of house, fixing windows and ventilation. It even proposed that one needs more space in the backyard than the front setback. This procedure helps vegetable and immediate herbal needs from the backyard too. If Vaastu purush is not happy, that house adds problems for the living person!

Observation XI: Fiscal discipline: The game of money- ever since it is being launched had a rationale in India. In India, finance was analyzed by Chanakya in his book Arth- Sastra (a financial order) several centuries ago. It is the money that moves the wheels of country's economy. Hence, rupee or rupiah as Mahatma calls it or as some consider it as- rooh-ka-pahiah (wheel of moving soul or Lakshmi),- is vital for circulation. Here again, the Indo-British cooperation had its way in introducing paper and coin mint & also its regulation. During the British rule one rupee is made equal to one silver tola and it is so pure one can directly use that coin in making of medicines.

This vital point is that the coins served as standard weight and purity of metal too- till 1957- wherein India had switched currency to metric mode.

At the time of Indian independence, Indian rupee was strong and even then- after 1967 forced devaluation by IMF, one dollar equals to 4.5 rupees and one mark equal to 3.3 rupees in 1980, which I exchanged during my foreign travel.

Old rupee divisions: What was the old Indian money and how it was given breakup then? Since moon has sixteen shades (starting from- no moon night to full moon night), the pious Goddess- Lakshmi also is in sixteen shades. Then 1/16th rupee was one anna (also, one anna is equal to four kani). There are sixteen ways to please

God which were also known as shodasa-upacha-ra. There are sixty-four variety of arts (4x16)- making 16/64 as vital numbers. Further, Rupee/anna/Beda (two anna)/Dabboo (1/3 anna or four old paisa) and even kani or old paisa (one kani equals to three paisa)- all were of standard weights in British rule.

In ayurveda, they used to weigh ayurvedic drugs. From that level, the present progress is that the coins lost their significance both as standard weights, standard sizes. Now, one rupee equals to 100 Naya-paise and 5, 10, & 20 paisa- mint replaced 16 anna structure of rupee.

Present day currency: In 1970, IMF delinked gold holdings to currency minting by any nation- a fundamental mistake. India objected and was never a member of ruling IMF- G8- later. IMF made space for even communist currencies, (with known for unlimited controls on minting,) thereby strengthening Russia & China.

The golden rule in original way of minting currency & bonds etc., is limited to five times the gold holding. This was given good bye and this paper currency causing severe inflation in many countries!

Observation XII: In mathematics, all count begins from zero. What is that zero? If Poornam-Adah to poornam--- added zero; Poornam-edam to poornam----multiplied with zero; Poornam subtracted (adaya) from poornam- still the answer is zero. Here, n + 0= n or n x 0=0 or n – 0 =n, all give the unique answer 0; and if n=0, still value do not change. It Is a sloka in Sanskrit, in puja!

Thanks to the recital memory of Sanskrit scholars who propagated orally. Hence, Sanskrit sloka are sanctum. There are many meanings for the same sloka and this needs a separate explanation through scholars.

Observation XIV: Without equipment-measurements:

1. In the British model, one pint, one pound (currency), one pound as weight and one fathom as distance, are standards- in a simple way! Here, Pint is the standard volume @ 473 ml of fluid and one fathom is the distance covered with both hands stretched by a man and it equals to 1.82 meters or two gajam. Probably, gajam or a giant step is the @distance covered by an elephant in one step.

2. In the whole sale market, weight of one man is @one tuta in Hindi- how potatoes and onions are still available. The next largest common weight then is thus one maund, which as defined by British is 37 kg. The next smaller weight is Dadi- in Hindi (5.5kg or roughly ¼ th cube foot stone or one Dadi = @four veesa in Telugu). Still lower denomination is one ounce or 28.35 grams wherein 16 ounces make one pound then.

Further, two anna= one kasu or savara or 8 gm. (Wherein- 11.664 gm. = one old tola); The lowest weight then was- one guri(venda)-ginja or Guriginja seed (3mg.)- that is the standard weight in old system. Still these seeds are used for weighing gold. I located that plant during my child-hood days on the top of Talupula amma-lova, near Tuni (AP). In 1980-when I purchased gold ornaments, I saw their use even in J&K. At present, 10 grams gold is treated as one tola – a simplification now.

3. The big commonly handled volume is one bag of rice grains called putty. It is divided into twenty kuncham. Here, one kuncham is equal to four ser. One ser equals to four sola & so on.

4. When the area is quantified, the unit is one Kunta or gunta (the area of land- irrigable- using a well)-i.e., (11x11)- 121 sq. yards and 40 gunta equal to one acre, thus 2.47 acres make one

hectare. Even now, one acre is 4840 sq. yards and one cent (metric nomenclature) is 48.4 sq. yards or 40.46 sq. meters & so on.

5. The British unit is mile- equal to eight furlongs. One furlong is equal to @20 guntha. One guntha is 11 yards or 10 meters or 33 feet. In measuring distances again, one gajam has two Maura. Maura (one elbow of man, @ 18") is equal to two Jaana. Each Jaana(a stretched distance covered from the tip of the thumb to the tip of little finger by hand).

One yojanam is a unit for longest distance in Sanskrit, like Amada in Telugu. Yojanam can be derived from the epic Ramayana – as the length of Ajodhya is twelve yojanam and width is three yojanam. The submerged Dwaraka was said to be of 12 yojanam long and its area is @80 yojanam. The reminiscent of Dwarka fort in sea was spread in @4 sq. km area that match with the Mahabharat descriptions. The final confirmation is in Ramayana, Sau Yojanam is the distance in sea between India & Sri Lanka and now it is known to be @70-80 kms.

Observation XIV (Money and Mahatma Gandhi): Given a difficult situation, how to survive? Mahatma Gandhi practiced austerity throughout his life and said to have maintained his diet to five paise/day in his ashram as that was the average Indian income during the British regime. Ayurveda is one of the health care systems & many books on medicinal systems available. There are more than thirty types of medicinal systems existed all over the world. The present Indian system is getting amalgamated under the ministry of AYUSH (Ayurveda, Yoga, Unani, Siddha, and Homeopathy-pooled into one system). I am somewhat familiar with magneto therapy; acupressure and yogic exercises in Yoga Sat sang classes-thanks to the training in allied medicine courses.

As someone holding a doctorate in natural chemistry, my inclination has always been toward unraveling the scientific underpinnings of traditional practices. Witnessing the tangible effectiveness of these remedies, coupled with my academic background, has ignited a fervent desire to explore and share their potential benefits with a broader audience.

May the pages of this book serve as a guiding light for readers in search of holistic approaches to wellness, weaving together the timeless wisdom of home remedies with the insights of modern science?

In essence, this book serves as a guiding light for readers seeking holistic approaches to wellness, weaving together the timeless wisdom of home remedies with the insights of modern science. May it inspire a deeper appreciation for the harmony between tradition and innovation in our pursuit of well-being.

Warm regards,

Dr. P Gangadhara Rao

Email: pgrao51@gmail.com

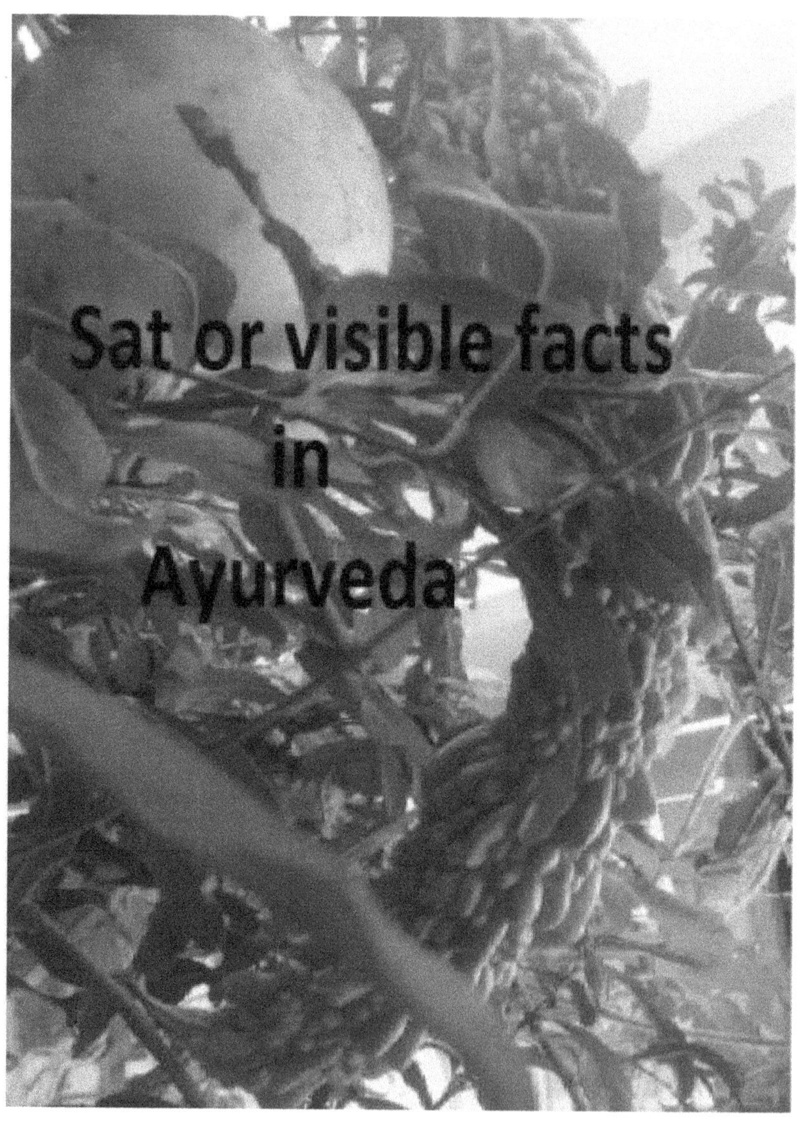

Karela creeper on pomegranate tree

Part - I

Health as Home Cure in First Five Chapters

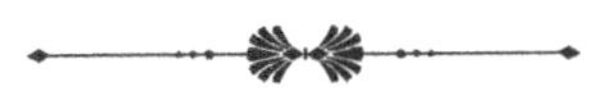

Idol Worship- as a curtain raiser: The earth, fire, water,air and sky – are the panca-mahabhoot &- sanctum. Any treatment (naturopathy) is possible through them. Thus, stay in high altitudes for fresh air (air), bathe in different springs and rivers as hydrotherapy (water), use of plant herb/spice in treating minor ailments (earth), use of cooked foods (fire) and even astrology (sky) – are used for improving health.

How our normal life and health is linked to the Idol worship? – Let us look into some procedural details to extract some information. The Idols (like Vishnu or Shiva or Rama or Durga or even Hanuman) are regularly decorated and worshipped every day with flowers, herbs, fruits or even with cooked food. The Idol becomes divine after installation with chanting mantra called prana-Protista (infusing life). The mantra suggests that the Idol is ritu- Sudarshan- kaal..iti….dikh-..bandha-ha. It means the idol like a human, needs cleaning, needs clothing, shelter, food (like a child), allowed to sleep and even married. In purusha-Suk- tam, the word used is "drusy-ate. sruyate."- which means God is ever watching & hearing each activity.

1. How worship begins?: It begins as- 'Om...A Pavitra-pavitropah.... sarva. Avastan. Gatoh. Pivah. Ye... Smaret ... Pundarika.- Akshah. – Sabahya...antarah ...suchi-hi'- It means – priest seeks permission to touch the Idol by saying- that I came through all stages of cleanliness before touching the lotus eyed God. So, not only taking bath is an essential, but also the Idol is to be bathed. How? – with clean water.

1.ii: Idol, bath & mantra:

"Gangaicha-... Yamunae. Cha... Godavari. Saraswathi, Narmadae. Sindhu. Kaveri.-"

Using waters of seven immortal rivers or clean lake water or well water we bathe you. How an Idol is given bath – is it only water? No, it is also bathed later with milk, curd, honey, ghee, fruit juice, coconut water, sandal paste, amla paste, black gram pastes and even turmeric/haldi paste etc., suggesting the people how can come out of diseases.

After the bath, the Idol is decorated with bilwa patra, tulasi, and fragrant flowers/garlands- courtesy plant and flower collectors or devotees. They are mostly fungicidal or bactericidal with rich fragrance. Lord Shiva is specially decorated with vibhuti (scented ash) also. Now-a-days people use talcum powder- after our bath. Is it not a scented calcined ash?

1. The Food & Mantra: In Lalita sahasram "Guda. Anna

..Preet a...Manase" – means Jaggery or Gur and cooked rice preferably with ghee- (called chakkera-pongal) is liked by Goddess. In suprabhatam, Lord Venkateshwara during wakeup call- in mantra is offered "kadali... Phala... paayasa" – means well-cooked kheer (rice, milk, dry fruits and jaggery) and with a fruit of banana is waiting for you to be served. Similarly, every commoner, after consuming food says 'ah- jaan-aagayee'.

How it is digested, the mantra suggests?

(Prana—Apana…vyanau-udana—samana.)-- means

A. "Om- Pranay- a swahah…-it is receiving life as food;

B. Om udanaya swahah… enters (Udara) stomach;

C. Om samanaya swahah…. food is leveled;

D. Om vyanaya swahah. Enters blood & also lower parts;

E. Om apanaya swahah. Digestive gas released;

F. Om brahmane swahah. Reached Brahma (the soul);

This happens naturally through the blood circulation in the order as above and these are covered as shodasha (-sixteen)- up achara (ways of serving) to the Idol. So, the Idol needs are exactly similar to the human needs like- cleaning, clothing & decoration (flower garlands) and offering food- all three major tasks are covered.

'Thus, worship procedure is nothing but the basic human needs – described as food, water, shelter & clothing.' The notion exists such as "roti kapadah-aur makaan"- means food, clothing and shelter.- is exactly the same.

1.iv: Food security: The staple foods in the old days are nine cereals – called nava- dhanya, with reproducible seeds for centuries. Indians managed using them for their food in survival.

In order to have a staple food, not only one needs good cultivatable land but also continuous water supply, plus-needs animals for farming. As a result, many races have settled in India as the land is "sujalam, sufalam and- malayaja-seetalam"- means, the land is rich in good water, fruits, cattle and healthy breeze. Lord shiva used Nandi (ox) as his vehicle.

1.v: Hydrotherapy: It is a general rule to take bath in the ponds near temples and Shrines, that exist mostly on the banks of rivers. In fact, all old cities in India or even abroad, were built on river banks. There are sulfur springs or hot water springs near some shrines that improve health. Hence, bathing in different waters for a long time is an automatic hydrotherapy. This removes clog from kidneys and abdomen through reverse osmosis. Even ponds/rivers help in reverse osmosis.

Thus, it is only good water – that can keep a person alive for a longer time. How to maintain a good water supply? In the Himalayas, many drops of melting snow make a stream, later many-rills, gullies & streams,- lead to form river(s).

These Himalayas host substantial water as ksheer Sagar Lake (Milk- like- lake or manas-Sarovar at the feet of the Mount – Kailash or home of Shiva). The noteworthy fact is that this lake & Himalayas account for Ganga, Yamuna, Brahmaputra, Sindh and many more rivers & tributaries.

These Himalayas account for nearly three billion human population (India, China, Nepal, Bhutan, Pakistan, Burma & Bangladesh) or nearly half humans living on earth. Here, Ganges, Brahmaputra, and Sindh are the mighty rivers with many tributaries. The longest river in India is Ganges which accounts for 36% of cultivated land in India, plus yields lot of fish at the Bay of Bengal, by absorbing Brahmaputra River flowing from China- up to west Bengal & Bangladesh!

Down South, there is another range of hills called Meruparvat (Vindhyachal), wherein the major rivers Narmada, Tapti, Godavari, Krishna and other tributaries like Tungabhadra, Kaveri and Penna- originate. They form major source of water to feed about 38 to 40% of the population in down south. Indians practice, worshipping one river each year. This matches with Jupiter's arrival nearer to earth- every year. Here, the planet earth completes one revolution – round the Sun in a year. Jupiter needs twelve years for one rotation round the Sun. Thus, Jupiter, the largest graham in Solar system- impacts earth- every year. It is worshipped as kumbha mela.Hence, river linked hydrotherapy is propagated through astrology. Ganga Pushkar happens when Guru (Jupiter) entering Mesha (Aries). Then following year, Narmada Pushkar in Rishabh (Taurus), Saraswathi in Mithuna (Gemini), Yamuna in Karka or Karkataka (Cancer), Godavari in Leo (Simha), Krishna in Kanya (Virgo), Kaveri in Tula (Libra), Bhima in Vrishchika (Scorpio), Tapti (also known as Pushkar-Vahini) in Dhanus (Sagittarius), Tungabhadra in Makara (Capricorn), Sindhu (Indus) in Kumbha (Aquarius), and finally Pranahita (Parineeti) in Pisces (Mina). Kumbha-mela signals-arrival of Brihaspati nearby & so time to fill kumbha (pond) in every village with water as all rivers are in spate then!

Further, so collected water remains fresh with flora and fauna- making eco- system-viable through the ponds. Means, the basic drinking water facility also exists for all throughout the year.

Hence, "aapovah. Edagam. Sarvam..." – means water is everything for survival. Thus, most of the world's famous old cities existed only on the river banks or near sea.

Simple mode of cure is through Sun-bath/and hydrotherapy. Swimming is also a best exercise and is an ideal hydrotherapy. Another is warm water plus salt (for curing itch in the feet) near

Sulphur springs, that exist near temples or keep feet in sea waters or even bath in sea waters. If one visits a shrine, he takes bath in a pond with priest chanting mantra. The reverse osmosis or hydrotherapy begins, provided ponds nearby the temples are clean with tortoise and fish!

1.vi: Festivals: Indian festivals, look like a farmer's calendar and the oldest teacher being Lord Shankar. Lord Shiva always held fresh water (Ganga) on his head and moved on ox- suggesting agriculture as the suggested profession. If one remembers a common saying in Hindi "uttam kheti madhyam vyapar……" suggesting- agriculture as the best profession. Shiva's wife is the daughter of the hill (Parvati), and also is known as Annapurna. She is worshipped all over India as she liberally provided food to all needy.

Similarly, the festival of Makara Sankranti (Beginning of Solar calendar) or Lohri is celebrated throughout India and it begins with offering of Chirwa, Rewari (sesame seeds plus Gur), groundnut, ghee and also some new crops to devta, through cow-dung & wood burnt fire. Animal also worshipped. It also declares the end of winter session and the cleaning work begins by throwing waste out of the houses. Some homes exhibition of all variety dolls – is a common practice.

The next is Vaisakhi festival, for wheat cutting and sowing summer crops; Durga festival before seed testing before sowing; Diwali for harvest of summer crops & fertilizer addition. It is followed by nag-chivithi so on.

Farmers do not kill snakes as they consume wild rats- protecting crops. On nag-pancami in some parts of India or Nagula chavithi-in AP, the snakes are worshipped and the mud brought from that place is applied to the ear.

This prevents deafness. How? One guruji said boil that mud in sesame oil, filter & use as ear drops. I prefer garlic oil as ear drops.

Food is taken care of- using renewable seeds of nava-dhanya.

Before ace crop in India, on Vijayadashami day, all cereals tested as shoots- offered to Goddess every year. It is also a seed testing vs soil.

1.vii: More from Idol worship?

1. In case you are static to a place like an Idol (dik bandha ha), there is a longer life. Further, if you are in a hilly area- life gets prolonged.

2. If you respire slowly,- the life gets prolonged. Tortoise is the longest living (four hundred years), with one respiration in four minutes, whale takes one respiration per minute (@100 years), man takes two respirations per minute (@50 years + medicine adds extra medical support).

3. A dog respires faster but lives @ 18 years & rabbits or rats live shorter so on. There is a saying that God inside us counts the number of respirations and ends the life when its count is over- like a computer. If one is respiring faster, (– except due to over exhaustion, or run/exercise)- his death is nearby. That's why people call- 'thand rakh'-/be cool.

4. There is a saying that man has to fight a disease and the medicine improves health. Faith on God brings additional support in your will power.

5. Temples generate work for plant, flower or fruit collectors and vendors. As in mantra, the basic necessities of an Idol are clean water, fresh leaves, clothes for decoration, and finally fruits.

Thus, the Idol worship means faith therapy, hydrotherapy & naturopathy.

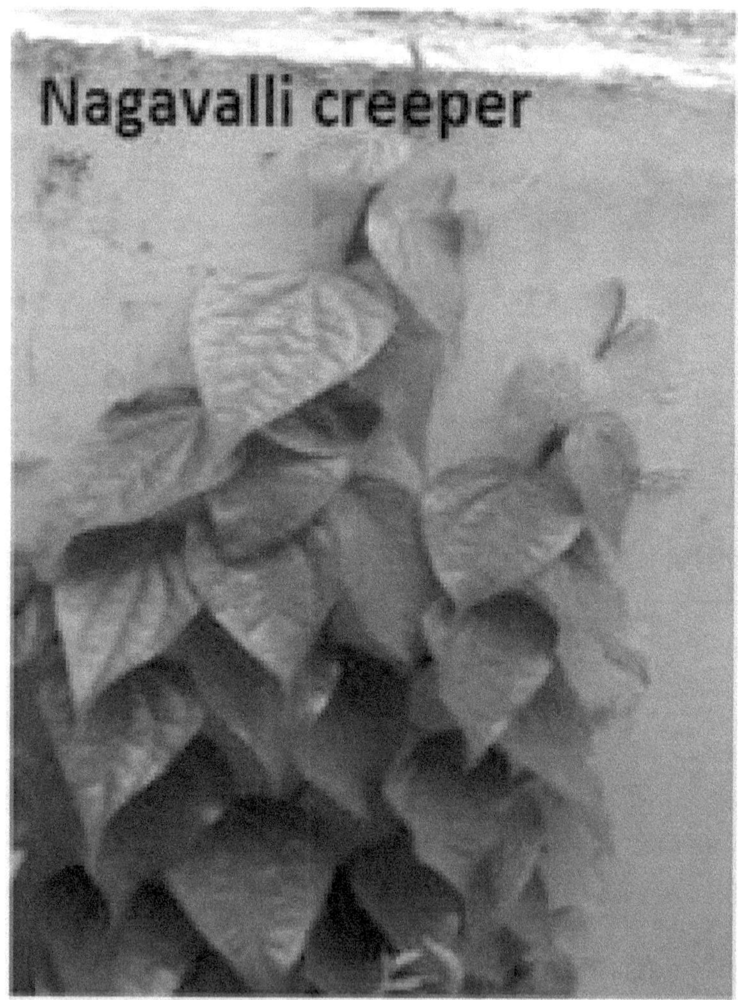

While every festival is linked to the farmer's calendar, only Ganesh puja is not so! Why?

See ganesh pjua.

2. Ganesh Puja

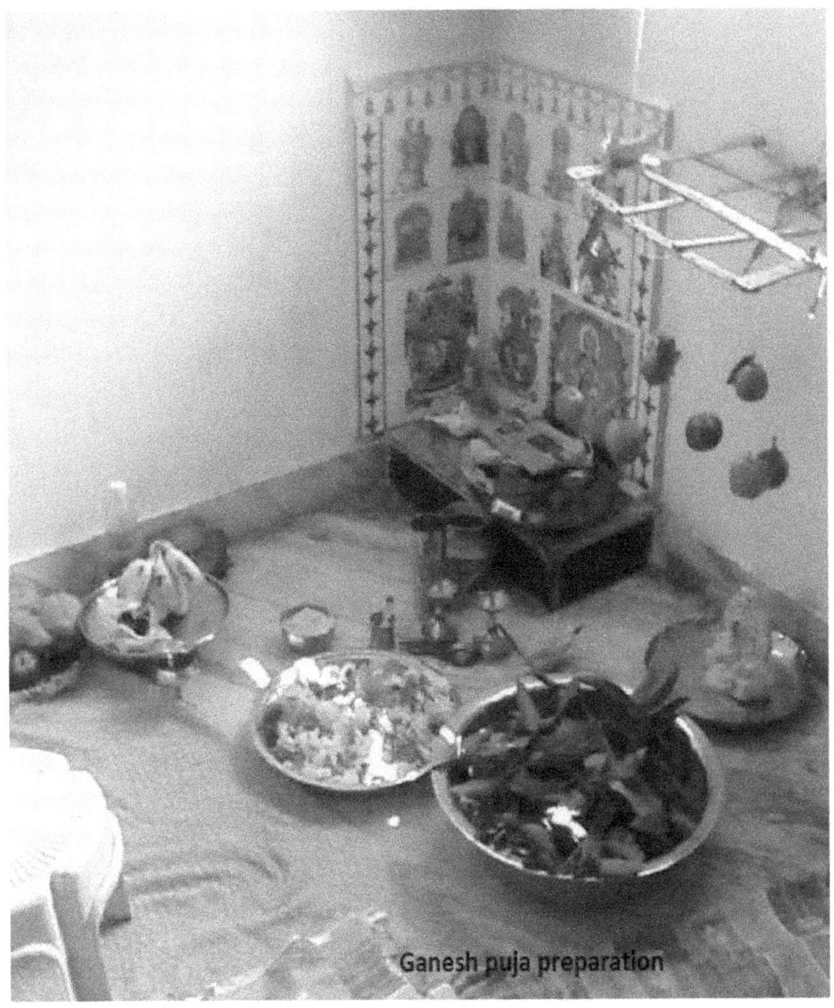

Photo1: preparation;

2.i. Significance of Ganesh Puja

The first and second sloka in Vishnu sahasra-namam pray Ganesh and also Hayagriva. These are one of the first Idols to be worshipped before beginning any work. Ganesh was created from mud and was given life by Parvathi, (the wife of Shiva). In fact, all creations are from mud, but we need panca-mahabhoot to bring Chaitanya into that soil.

A. Before beginning any new work, one should be humble and thus bow the head before the God (or Boss) to achieve success. Hence, before start of every work, God is to be appeased. Same is done even today- by calling big Boss for inauguration or ribbon cutting!

B. What is the significance of the puja? Ganesh is not a born king. He is one among us who rose to supremacy on his own efforts. Ganesh had thus established control over siddhi and buddhi. Hence, he is an appointed leader & settled as an obstacle remover. So, he is head of armed forces (Ganapathy) or Vishwa-nayaka (world leader).

C. When faced with allegations, even Lord Krishna remembered Ganesh for clarity in thoughtful actions to be taken- it means Ganesh is a good adviser. Later Krishna puts all efforts towards a solution and it is his investigative journalism that led to the solution- called Samantaka-upakhyanam,- a lesson to remember by every person in crisis.

D. On the selected day for puja or around that period, there exists maximum greenery even to feed a herd of elephants. Once, Ganesh overate & ended up with stomach burst (diarrhea). This is a corollary- during the rainy season diarrhea- as a pandemic is hinted through the puja. To prevent such ill effects, use vavilli herb collected for puja.

E. Most plant collections are programmed in such a way that even children are tuned to locate the correct plant from the childhood. Before collection, any plant material needs a thorough identification like leaf, stem, flower bud, fruit and seed structures, which are characteristic of every plant. Ganesh puja time is exactly coined to such herb collection.

F. Ganesh puja brings in lot of peace and prosperity- as Chair is one and there are many competent (like Shanmukh) to be satisfied. Ganesh is always pleasing & with a steady mind. Leader should be non-revengeful- another point that is to be remembered by the new chair occupants.

G. Ganesh is a good listener- like an elephant which recognize voices from @50- 70 kms. Ganesh understood Mahabharat thoroughly and wrote to the exact dictates of Vyasa mahamuni as he is the fastest writer too. Corollary: A boss should be a good listener, less talkative, intelligent, majestic and brisk mover & all such properties amply exist with an elephant!

H. Even, Ganesh's rat also has a history and is called a-nindya or non- problematic. Here, like an active rat cutting roots- our mind continuously pokes something into the brain!

I. Why that day chosen for puja?- On that day, the star galaxy looks like an elephant tusk (Hasta formation) or like an extended palm on that day- every year,- means astral blessing is also asserted.

J. Ganesh/animal heads/decorated demons/use shapes of animals or snakes or ghost heads or Dracula etc., as local traditions- displayed in many parts of the world starting from Japan, China, Germeany & even USA. In Germany, I saw one such mass extravaganza in summer fest with peculiar shapes worn by the public in that display.

2.ii. How to do Puja

It is done in a neat selected & decorated place for puja (as shown in page 26). It needs 21 plant varieties of fresh leaves for puja. The methods of appeasement suggested for Ganesh are patram (leaves for elephant, i.e., food), pushpam (flowers), phalam (sweets and fruits) and toyam (gifts/flower garlands)- that is true even today!

2. ii. a. AP Region Plants

This region was called tri-linga-desa. Later this region is called Telugu speaking land, called Andhra Pradesh (Besides AP, Telangana, parts of Odisha and Chhattisgarh- are Telugu speaking too). Ganesh is prayed in these regions, with leaves of herbs like- Arjuna pat-ram (tellamaddi), Apamarga patram (Uttareni), Arka patram (jilledu), Asvattha patram (Ravi), Bilva-patram (maredu), Badari patram (regu), Brihati-patram (vakudu), Chuta patram (mamidi), Dadimi patram (danimma), Datura patram (ummetta, unmatta- is self-explanatory), Durva-yugmam (Garrika), Also, Devadaru patram (deodar), Gandaki patram (devakanchanam), Jaji patram (jaji), Karavira patram (ganneru), Machi patram (machipatri), Maruvaka patram (maruvam), Sami patram (jammi), Sindhuvara patram (vavilli), tulasi patram (tulasi), Vishnukanta patram (vishnukanta). Velaga fruit: Feronia limonida/F. elephantum or kaith or wood apple or kapittha or velaga fruit offered. Its leaves are aromatic, carminative, bark cure biliousness (recommended too); fruit astringent, stimulant, stomachic & acidic. This fruit is considered to be the hot favorite for Ganesh.

2.ii.b. Maharashtra Region Plants

Also worships with medicinal herbs that are slightly different from AP herbs, they are, aghada, apta, Arjun, Ashok, Brahmi, Bael, Bor,

Durva, Dalimb, Devadaru, Dhotra, Dorli, Hadga, Jaye, Jaswand, Kewda, Kanher, Marva, Madhu-malathi, Madar, Maka, Nir-gundi, Peepal, Sami, Tulas, & vishnukanta. After doing all the worship with leaves and grass, the final is a steam cooked food offered to Ganesh and along with a pan (Naga Valli dalairyutam--- Mukta – churnena samyuktam – tambulam. prati-gruhyatam...) a betel leaf on which thin layer of calcium coated along with more supplements of pan like supari-added & folded. Then, it is offered. The studies in Sweden confirm that calcium helps in the insulin release. Supari helps in the breaking of old blood cells to form bile and bilirubin-is well known! Finally, camphor- burnt as arati which spreads fragrance that kill bacilli & it completes the puja.

2.iii: The Final List of Herbs

Some AP plants differ from Maharashtra region and the sum total of them gives a good list of herbs. It will be given after puja celebrations for Ganesh. During the puja, with the mantra- the selected leaves are as below.

1. Om sumukhaya namah, Machi-patram samarpayami: Artemisia vulgaris or Artemisia indica, Mug wort; an infusion of leaves is used in the treatment of nervous and spasmodic affections, in asthma and in diseases of the brain. This infusion is an appetizer. The juice of the plant is used in Nepal to treat diarrhea, dysentery and abdominal pains. Its oil used to cure earache and its paste is an external cure for boils and injuries. Whole plant is an emmenagogue, anthelmintic, antiseptic, and stomachic too.

2. Om ganadhipa-yanamah: Brihati patram samarpayami: Solanum indicum, Vakudu, Nightshade: Bir-Hathi is also its name in old texts. It means bad is avoided. Its root is carminative,

expectorant, and useful in asthma, cough, catarrh, toothache, and cures fevers. The alkaloids solanine, solasodine are present in leaf and root. It is and a liver tonic cures indigestion also. But it grows in high altitudes only.

However, in warmer part of India, the other species grow wild. Some are:

Ranvangi, Solanum Surettence, Brihati, Dorli, Ranvangi, Vakudu, – root is carminative, expectorant, useful in asthma, cough, catarrh, toothache and even fevers. Leaves as poultice cure itch. Nelamulaka, Solanum xanthocarpum (syn S. surettence) and other species grow down southern India & is considered hepato-protective, anti-inflammatory, antitumor, diuretic, and antipyretic;

3. Om gauriputraya namah: or Om umaputraya namah: Bilva patram samarpayami: Aegle marmelos, Bilva, Maredu, Sri phal, Shiva's food, Bael, Bilwa; unripe fruit pulp is astringent, digestive, stomachic & good for health; Ripened fruit is aromatic, cooling and laxative; Root bark cures intermittent fevers; unripe fruit is astringent, digestive, & stomachic; It reduces impact of poisons. It contains marmeloin (imepitoin), also umbelliferon & others.

4. Om Gajananaya namah: Durvara patram samarpayami: Cynodon dactylon, Durva, Common grass; its infusion of the root used for stopping bleeding piles; poultice fresh cuts and wounds; internal used in catarrh, and ophthalmic to wash eyes. According to Unani system of medicine, it is used as a laxative, coolant, and expectorant, carminative and as a brain and heart tonic. In Homoeopathic systems of medicine, it is used to treat all types of bleeding and skin troubles.

5. Om harasunave namah: Datura patram samarpayami: Datura stramonium or D. metel (Ummetta, Dhotra); Its name seems to me is evolved out of unmatta- meaning drowsy, which later became ummetta. Thus, it cures cerebral complications, besides asthma or bronchitis in internal consumptions and externally for joint pains. Its leaves, seeds, roots in fact all cure fevers, catarrh.

6. Om Lambodaraya namah: Badari patram samarpayami: Ziziphus marutiana/Z. jujube, Gangaregu, Bor: It cures throat infection; fruits externally are used to remove bad omen; internally mucilaginous, pectoral, styptic and blood purifier; bark is anti-diarrheal. It is available as saltish chakki (fruit, spice and salt dried) for regular consumption throughout the year.

7. Om Guha-agrajaya namah: Apamarga patram samarpayami: Achyranthes aspera, Uttareni, Aghada, Prickly chaff; used in dropsy, piles, boils, skin eruptions, and colic, used in scorpion or snake bite; infusion of roots astringent and seeds emetic; Its seeds boiled and consumed with rice to increase quality of male fertility. Its leaf oil cures ear related problems.

8. Om gajakarnaya namah: or Om gajakarnikaya namah: Tulasi patram samarpayami: Ocimum sanctum, Ocimum tenuiflorum, Tulasi, Tulas, Holy Basil: It is sweet Stomachic, anthelmintic, diaphoretic, expectorant, antipyretic, carminative, stimulant, diuretic, demulcent, in asthma, and ophthalmia. It's almost all parts, like leaf, stem, flower, root, seeds are used for the treatment of bronchitis, malaria, diarrhea, dysentery, skin disease, arthritis, eye diseases, insect bites and so on.

9. Om ekadantaya namah: Chuta patram samarpayami: Mangifera indica (Mamidi, Amra): leaves astringent and useful

in uterine hemorrhages, also applied as poultice on scorpion sting; mango tree gum used to cure broken feet. Ripe fruit laxative, diuretic and delicious even and used for making jelly; unripe fruit is useful in ophthalmia and also on eruptions; seed kernel is useful in asthma & is a source of cocoa; cooked as vegetable; Its delicate shoots consumed to cure diarrhea; bark or chawl of the tree is astringent and useful in hemorrhages; Its leaf, stem, raw fruit, ripe fruit and even its seed is a medicine.

10. Om Vikataya namah: Karavira patram samarpayami: Thevetia nerifolia or Nerium oleander (Ganneru, Kanher); It is poisonous plant and flowers used in worship. It converts white hair to black and also prevent hair loss. root bark is crushed and its extract is made into oil & this oil is used for application on all skin diseases including leprosy; seeds are rich in amygdalin a cardiac depressant; It treats boils and injury healer externally & internally kernel is fatal, used in suicide.

11. Om Chinnadantaya namah: Vishnukantapatram samarpayami: Evolvulus alsinoides, Sankhapuspi: dried leaves smoked a cigarette for chronic bronchitis and asthma; it improves nerve strength and also help in memory retention cures mental disturbances; applied on boils.

12. Om vatave namah: Dadimi patram samarpayami: Punica granatum (Anar, Danimma, Dalimb); Cures anemia, cures piles, root & stem bark are astringent, anthelmintic, and specific tape worm killer; Anar- root and stem bark extracts are used as astringent and it is tapeworm elimination. Cures diarrhea and dysentery; Fruit pulp is cardiac and stomachic & recommended diet in fevers. Its dried seed is known as source of acid- used in sore throats, coughs, urinary infections, digestive

disorders. Dried rind of fruit, along cloves cures diarrhea and dysentery; Prevents nasal bleeding.

13. Om sarveswaraya namah: Cedrus deodar: Devadarupatram samarpayami: diaphoretic, carminative, used in fevers, flatulence, urinary disorders & piles, gravels in kidney, and considered as antidote to snake bite; an injury healer, and also skin diseases. Bark astringent, used in fevers, diarrhea and dysentery.

14. Om phalachandraya namah: Maruvaka patram samarpayami: Origanum Majorana (Maruvam, Marjoram, Marzano's, Marumam, Marva, Marwa); Maruvam is used for joint pains, cures vata diseases, cures cough and also heart related diseases. It is a good general tonic, used for-digestive and respiratory systems. Dhavanam/Artemisia pallens is a plant carminative, expectorant, and tonic; the leaves & seeds are astringent, remedy to colic, liver stimulant and antispasmodic.

15. Om Herambhaya namah: Sindhuvara patram samarpayami: Vitex negundo (Nir gundi or Nalla vavilli or Saraswathi leaf); used for catarrh, fever, heaviness of head and dullness in hearing; drie d leaf is smoked to relieve catarrh and also intermittent fevers and headaches; leaf powder as paste used for dispensing swelling joints and acute rheumatism; It reduces impact of poison. It reduces body pains and cures vata related problems.

16. Om surpakarnaya namah: Jaji patram samarpayami: Jasminum grandiflorum, Chambeli, Adavimalli, Chamoli Jasminum officinale, Yasmeen, Jasmine: Fragrant flowering plant and its whole plant (wp) is anthelmintic, diuretic, emmenagogue; wp paste used externally to cure allergies; wp ext. contains mixtures

of coumarins, cardiac glycosides, essential oils, flavonoids, phenolics and saponins etc.; juice of leaves applied on corns, poured into ears to cure otorrhea; leaves chewed and spitted out for curing mouth ulcers, the plant is anthelmintic, diuretic, emetic.

17. Om Suragrajaya namah: Gandaki patram samarpayami: There is no plant as Gandaki, however, Gandana is there. But locals use the following plants. Bauhinia racemosa (Apta) preferred in Maharashtra or Bauhinia purpurea (Devakanchanam, Gandra); preferred in AP. Bauhinia purpurea, is a flowering plant is used in several traditional medicinal systems and known since ages. It cures various diseases & has been known to possess antibacterial, antidiabetic, anti-inflammatory, anti-diarrheal, anti-cancerous, analgesic, nephroprotective and thyroid hormone regulating activity. It is substituted for Gandaki patram. Apta, Bauhinia racemosa; is anti-oxidant and hepato- protective, refrigerant, astringent and is used in the treatment of headache, fever, skin diseases, blood diseases, dysentery and cleaning of ulcers. Beedi making leaf also has a commercial market.

My unique preference is for gandana as there is no plant Gandaki. Gandana, Achillea millefolium, Milfoil, Yarrow, Woundwort, Achilles heel, Soldier's woundwort, Rojmari: whole plant is emmenagogue, bloodwort, used as tea with fresh leaves like hypericum, injury healer, emollient; Europe & high altitudes, plant available. A folk medicine, chamazulenes rich; Used in chronic ulcers or external injuries, in inflammation and gastrointestinal disorders. It was known through Achilles — called Achilles heel for stanching the flow of blood from wounds and even called Soldier's wort. It is anti-tumor, cyto-protective, anti- nflammatory, analgesic, antioxidant, anti-microbial, hypotensive, Vaso protective, broncho dilatory, antispasmodic, and hepatoprotective too. It contains carbohydrates, organic acids, unsaturated fatty acids, tocopherols and phenolic acids also. Plant exists both in red or white flowers, both plants effective, but grow in moderately high altitudes-available in Himalayas.

18. Om ibhavaktraya namah: Sami patram samarpayami: Prosopis cineraria, Prosophis spicigera (Sami, Jammi, and Bannimara): If its chawl (beradu) is applied on to the skin, undesired hair is prevented. It cures breathing problems; Its pods are astringent and bark extract a remedy for rheumatism; flowers are powdered and consumed with sugar for womb retention; ash of the plant is rubbed all over the skin as it acts as hair remover.

19. Om Vinaya-kaya namah: Aswatha patram samarpayami: Ficus religiosa (Ravi, Pipal, Aswatha, Bodhi, Pippala, Peepul, Buddha); peepal or pippala is an astringent plant. See in Ficus species.

20. Om surasevitaya namah: Arjuna patram samarpayami: Terminalia Arjuna- is known as tellamaddi. See later in pages.

21. Om Kapila-ya namah: Arka patram samarpayami: Jilledu, Calotropis gigantea, Calotropis procera, Rui, Madar- is different names for this plant. People use the bark and root for medicine. Despite serious safety concerns about its extract blocking eyesight, its seeds float in air and hence called Rui.

Its leaf applied oil on one side, heated with haldi on the other side on frying pan and applied the oily side, after cooling on the joints and tied with muslin for a day. It relieves cramps and joint pains; cures parasitic infections externally including elephantiasis and worms. It is a diaphoretic, expectorant, and emetic. Powdered flowers useful in clod, asthma, cough and even indigestion.

Thus, this plant, flowers, roots all put together is known to cure more than fifty diseases. But it is highly poisonous and dangerous extract for the eyes also;

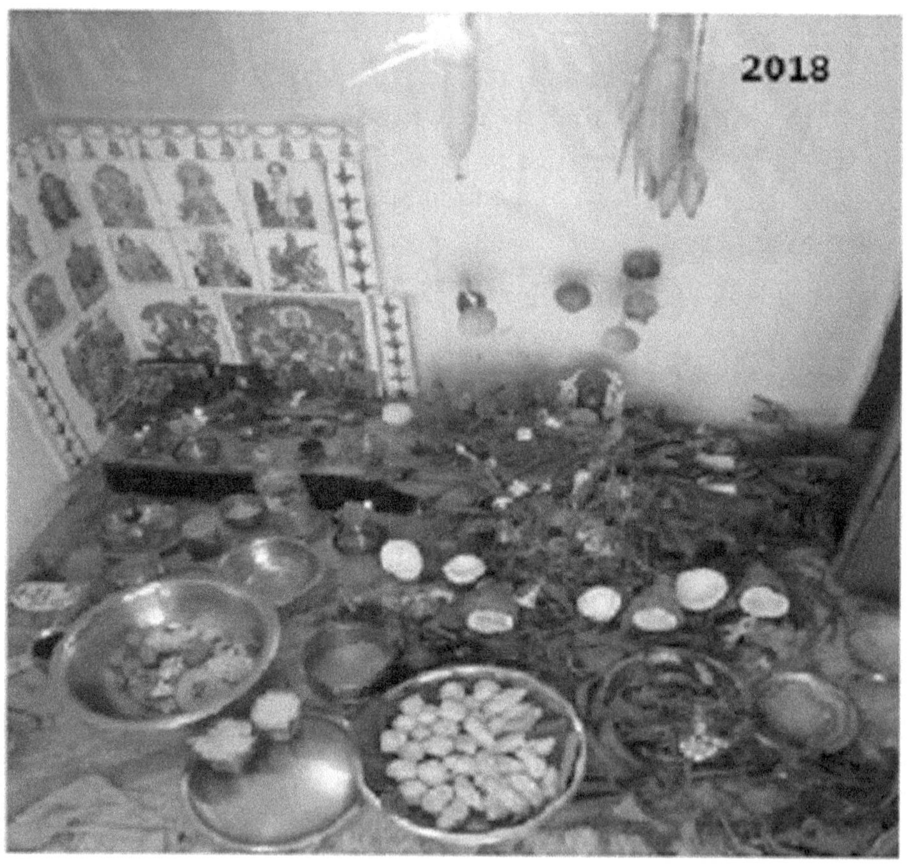

2: after puja

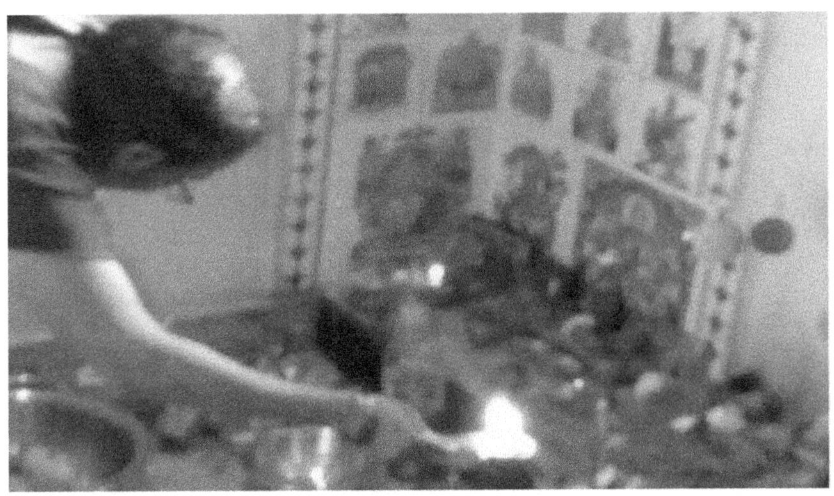

3: arati

Thus, we have offered all 21 variety leaves- mean you have a stock of all variety leaves for one year!

Here are more plants that added due to regional differences. There is nothing wrong if other herbs are also added for puja.

22. In South India there is no Deodar, Erythroxylon monogynum (bastard sandal) is substituted devadaru, but, of limited use. However, Asoka, Saraca asoca (uterotonic) is also called debdar in Bengali language and has all medicinal properties and uterotonic too-but not in this list. It is discussed below.

Sita Ashok or Saraca indica is known as debdar in Bengali. Ashok is a medicinal plant widely used in Ayurveda to treat painful conditions, improves complexion of the body, improves digestion and assimilation, alleviates excessive thirst, to kills all infectious agents, in blood disease, inflammation and also as CNS depressant, bark astringent; used in uterine affections; bark contain catechol, tannins, flavonoids, saponins, glycosides, steroids, phenolic compound and alkaloids., thus coolant. Its cut branch deteorates fast and even catch fungus. Hence is to be cleaned and dried fast in Sun. Asoka, Polyalthia longifolia,- which is also has uterotonic activity. It is stable and do not catch fungus after cutting. However, chuta patram in Ganesh puja, is the most widely available & safest emmenagogue.

23. Citrus Limonium (Jambira, gajanimma) is preferred in AP. Jambira, Citrus Limonium, Gajanimma; its fruit, juice, and peel- are used to make medicine. Lemon is used to treat scurvy, a condition caused by not having enough vitamin C. Lemon is also used for the common cold and flu, ringing in the ears (tinnitus), stomach upset and vomiting from pregnancy etc.

24. Agni Mantha, Clerodendrum Phlomidis, Arni, Arani, Takkolamu, Jai, Jaye, is preferred in Maharashtra. It is used in many popular therapies and its medicinal properties include inflammation, diabetes, nervous disorder, asthma, rheumatism, digestive disorders, and urinary disorders as well as a bitter tonic. Root is bitter tonic and given in convalescence of measles. Juice of leaves is alterative and given in neglected syphilitic complaints.

The root is given as a demulcent, & helps cure stomach troubles and swellings in cattle. A variety of constituents have been isolated and characterized from this genus including monoterpene and it's derivatives, terpenoids, and flavonoid glycosides, phenyl-ethanoic glycosides, steroids and steroid glycosides, etc.

25. Sesbania grandiflora, Agasti, Hadga, avese chettu, Agastya- is also a reputed medicinal plant – preferred in Maharashtra. Agastya is the star that comes in Sharad ritu in Indian calendar. This plant blooms in that period and hence is also known as "Agathi" plant. All parts of this plant are of medicinal value.

    Agasti leaves and flowers are used to improve digestive strength. It is also used to treat intestinal worms. Leaf paste is chewed to treat oral and throat infections. Bark is useful in treating the diarrhea. The leaves, pods and flowers are used in cooking for making delicious recipes.

    Paste of Agastya root and bark is applied externally to relieve pain and also inflammation associated with arthritis or gout or rheumatism. (Here shallaki is a better substitute, discussed elsewhere) Powdered bark is applied in scabies ulceration of tongue and alimentary canal.

    Nasya of Agastya leaf juice extract dried – sucked into nose as nasya to cure headache. Plant also cures cough, fever, epilepsy. Its roots of roots of red flowered Agasthi and Datura stramonium are applied on painful swellings. Flowers are used to treat night blindness. The wood of Agastya plant is used for domestic purpose and used like bamboo in furniture.

26. Brahmi, Bacopa monnieri- has been used by Ayurvedic medical practitioners for centuries for a variety of purposes, including improving memory, reducing anxiety, and treating epilepsy. In fact, some research confirmed that it may boost brain function and alleviate anxiety and stress, among other benefits. Maharashtra prefers it. Lower effective version is vishnukranta-discussed already.

27. Pandanus facicularis (kevda, kewda, kevra) – preferred in Maharashtra. It is also used in Ayurveda to provide symptomatic relief in diabetes, fever, joint pain, earache and to manage threatened abortion as well as psychiatric conditions. Kewra is also used as a food flavor and in aromatic industry. Ketaki, Umbrella tree, Pandanus odoratissimus, Kewra, Kewda, Screw-pine; has been traditionally known as one of the Indian ayurvedic herb, used in diabetes, fever, joint pain, earache and in medicines to provide symptomatic relief in threatened abortion.

It cures psychiatric conditions, rheumatism, spasm, cold, flu, epilepsy, wounds, boils, scabies, ulcers, colic, hepatitis, syphilis, cancer as well as a cardiotonic, antioxidant, and aphrodisiac. Its distillate of pandanus flower water, can be used by the teaspoon in diluted form, as a food flavor and in aromatic industry.

28. Eclipta Alba is known as Maka, Trailing eclipta, False Daisy, Kesha raj, Bhringaraj, Guntagalagara and is a preferred in Maharashtra. It has been used in ayurvedic medicine for being a liver tonic and having beneficial effects on diabetes, eye, health, and hair.

Thus, it treats dandruff and dry scalp, prevents graying of hair, reduces baldness, helps in hair growth and prevents hair- fall. Its other names are Karisalankanni, Bhringraj, False daisy & Eclipta prostrata. It is also used like its predessor & used in similar way.

29. Feronia elephantium/F. acidissima fruit: Some persons suggest Velaga fruit as the best fruit for offering Ganesh. It has a good medicinal value too and is preferred in Andhra

Pradesh. This wood apple scientifically is known as Limonia Acidissima, Feronia Elephantum, Feronia Limonia, Hesperethusa Crenulata, Schinus Limonia, and local names include Kaitha, Curd fruit, Elephant apple, Monkey fruit, Wood apple, velaga, and Kaith etc. Its therapeutic benefits include anti-allergic, anti-bacterial and it has been utilized as traditional medicine.

Drinking wood apple fruit juice has several benefits for the stomach and digestive system. It is also known to be a good remedy for constipation and helps relieve discomfort. It helps in curing digestive problems like dysentery and diarrhea. It is anti-cancer too.

Thus, a summation of the two or three states yielded more choice for puja. A noteworthy point is that if the neighboring states differ in the list of 21 herbs, what will happen if at all – all regions of India submit their preferences? This is how probably the Indian Pharmacopoeia consisting of important plants was evolved for the nation.

2.iv: Use of Ganesh Puja Herbs

Based upon their activities, the herbs of Ganesh puja can be summarized as below.

Anthelmintic: machipatri, dadima, Sindhu Vara, for internal use and sannajaji for external use.

Antiseptic: machipatri, dhattura, durva, apamarga – all internal and Arjuna bark ash external.

Anti-asthmatic: machipatri, brihati, Sindhu Vara, arka flowers.

Anti-diarrheal: adari, dhattura, vishnukranta, dadima – rind of the fruit powder or its stem even, besides fruit.

Astringent: uttareni roots, amra, dadima, devadaru bark; maruvaka leaves and seeds, Arjuna bark.

Boils and ulcers: Nir-gundi, amra, devadaru, kara-Vira, jaji, and apamarga.

Cough and cold cure: arka, brihati for catarrh, amra leaf ext. and Sindhu Vara for catarrh.

Cardio tonic: dadima fruit pulp, Arjuna bark ext., amra fruit pulp, dudhi WP as tea.

Dropsy/bowel/spleen, liver troubles, diaphoretic, stomachic: Machipatri leaves on liver, badari fruit, maruvaka seeds & wp, dadima fruit, brihati even stop vomiting, besides above; Diseases of the brain including hysteria: machipatri, durva, Dhattura, Vishnukanta.

Emmenagogue: amra leaf ext. tonic, Nir gundi disease curative, aswatha- anti-implantation, Sami (jammi) flowers-womb retention.

Piles cure: kara-Vira, jaji, apamarga & Nir gundi.

Rheumatism/swellings: Nir gundi, devadaru oil, arka, apamarga for hydrocele internal, arka in old days used for elephantids externally.

Skin eruptions/itch cure/cuts/bruises: sannajaji flowers external, dhattura external, apamarga external, kara Vira root/bark external, aswattha bark both internal and external.

Strangury: badari leaf-stem paste as poultice.

Vermifuge: Nir gundi and Vishnukanta as febrifuge also

Fevers: brihati, bilwa, maka, devadaru bark, arka, & Agastya. In my opinion, Andrographis paniculatus (kalmegh) is an ideal choice.

Thus, our ancestors recommended the Ganesh festival probably for the collection of medicinal plant leaves. If such medicinal plant flowers are used for worship on regular basis, can there be a failure in recognition of a plant or can there be a shortage for medicines?

2.v: Mythology and Lessons

Here, one story is worth mention. Even during the Ramayana days, Rama and Lakshmana were rescued by herbs in time. Lord Krishna used to wear chengalva poodanda (flower garland – that shreds skin diseases). Coming even to the present day, the God-Vydyanath (shiva) or Goddess Durga- in many states- hold medicinal plant gardens useful for treatment.

Since these are God driven gardens that people rarely steal. For a healthy person, the herbs of Ganesh puja are significant as they can resist onset of any disease. Chhatrapati Shivaji's mother also used Ganesh puja in a massive scale and after ten days-Ganesh idol is submerged into the sea- which is still a tradition. It means this festival has long roots.

Ganesh puja has more to teach us. Here, Ganesh is brought home for puja, given a place worshipped with all good faith and received boons from him. Yet, after the worship, he is dissipated along with his chair into waters- suggesting, the body is short lived. A chair is temporary, while all his deeds are permanent'. Further, when chair is lost, by superannuation or supersession or death, the head (the ruler) is changed. Here, there are some real instances wherein some bureaucrats needed doctor's counsel – resulting in the use of psycho-tropic drugs.

If one remembers, janma. Mrityu. Jara… vyadhi. (The four sorrows namely- birth, death, ageing, diseases) are inevitable.

Thus, Ganesh is immersed into waters – suggesting change of guard every year. If one realizes these facts, change of leader proceeds is in a smooth way.

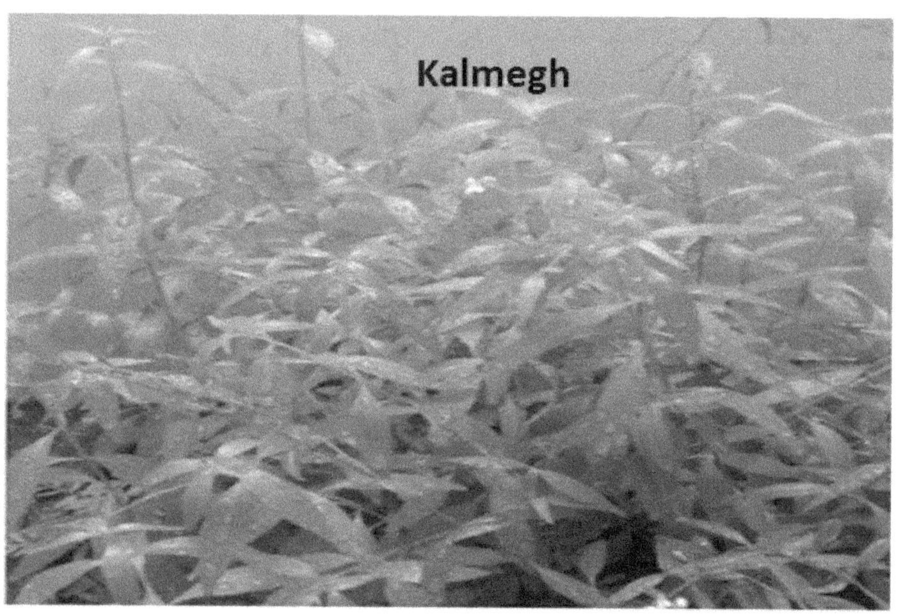

Kalmegh – grown at home;

3. Home Therapy

Once, I over-ate and physician gave an injection of siquil and asked me, 'did you find any fasted man dying early'?- Even fast unto death people did not die even after thirty days- that is the capacity of the body in furthering our survival. But an overloaded can die early.

Later, I opted fasting for about a week and I felt pain in stomach. So, I broke the fast. Then one yogi suggested me to keep fresh distilled water for fasting as salts from bore well cause the problem. This is the reason why maximum yogi or sanyasi live on Himalayas as that water is clean and practically salt less.

Vegan: Here, I call Vegan group-a luxurious class of people & only possible in warmer climates. If animal consumers do not exist, vegan group will be left with no grass or vegetable. Vegan group have lesser health problems also. In my opinion, the body has basically three enemies, one salt, the second excess oil use and finally, the third over-eating to be avoided. Animal food at some stage as one grows older also must be reduced. Excess food leads to lethargy and sluggish liver, – a known phenomenon.

Fast: Now, I never fast, but stopped overeating. The best way to fast as suggested by M. Satyanarayana Raju- a natural therapy specialist- proposed better options in fasting like-take lemon with honey after every two hours during the daytime. It ensures liver activation & fat digestion within the body.

An injured animal like,- dog or deer fasts for recovery in a corner or in a bush. But, when comes to us, fasting is done only during Ram-Navaratri and Devi-Navaratri — means for about ten days with cooked potato and little salt, or milk and banana- fasting- is most common. Another is Shivratri – Jagran, Mata-jagaratra, Vikuntha Ekadashi fasting etc. fast- are common. Taking one meal a day by Ayyappa devotees for forty days or fasting in Ramadan is still common. In good old days, fasting is recommended for every fever.

Coming into the subject, what one needs to do is tooth cleaning first. How?

3.a. Clean Teeth

i. Thus, choose one plant for your needs, now pickup natural teeth cleaner. My age-old preference is for cow dung – ash as tooth powder. My late father's preference is for vegetable coal power & rock salt. Tooth pastes can be made of babul, miswak or dantkanti, or Colgate herbal etc., or herbal twigs are readily available now. A herbal powder/& cow dung ash, mixed with salt/tingly herbs like mint oil and sorbitol transforms into an excellent tooth paste,- that is marketed.

Alternatively, Azadirachta indica (Neem tree), twigs if chewed for brushing teeth, it removes bad breath, protect gums & relieve toothache. Another is Salvadora persica or the toothbrush tree is a small evergreen tree native to India. Its sticks are traditionally used as a natural toothbrush called miswak, also known as salt brush, tooth brush tree, piludi, etc. names.

Before my home, I grew kami trees that provides tooth cleaning twigs forever. Cleaning teeth is a process that fights gum disease, prevents teeth decay & protect enamel on the teeth.

Babool (details): Nalla-tumma, Acacia Arabica, Vachellia nilotica, Gum Arabic, Keekar, Gum tree, Peet Pushpa- find more uses. The bark is cooling, astringent, demulcent, and anthelmintic. It also cures skin diseases. It prevents bleeding piles, and useful in diabetes. The decoction of this plant cures leucorrhea. It is useful in asthma and bronchitis. It is a good remedy to prevent hair fall, ear ache, syphilis, cholera, dysentery, leprosy and render-pest. bark astringent; gum, bark-demulcent, anti-diabetic; contain 40% tannins fruit.

The leaf poultice has good effect on bruises, infection and itch. Acacia Arabica contains gallic acid, m-di-gallic acid, catechin, chlorogenic acid, and also gallolyated flavan-3, 4-diol and robidandiol. The whole plant as a paste also relieves in hot inflammations.

Bleeding gums: Take lemon flowers and grind to paste and apply to teeth gums. It prevents correcting bleeding gums. Take onion paste and wash teeth with it, it also prevents bleeding of gums. Take black-vavilli leaf paste, camphor and white pepper all grinded to paste and kept in mouth by the side of teeth, again it eliminates bleeding gums. Take mehndi leaf paste of the size of senaga ginja (sabot chana size) with milk and applied thrice a day, to cure gums.

Bath: For taking a bath, oil is applied on the skin, later sunnipindi paste (mash and moong dal power in warm water) is applied, wait for ½ hr. and rub the skin thoroughly to eliminate dried paste and oil is my childhood method & using froth of soap-nut fruits, once a week complete bath was practiced. Of course, daily bath was a routine.

i. The Soap-nut (details): Arisaka, Soap-nut- Saponaria officinalis, Saponaria vaccaria, Sapindas Mukorossi and Sapindas Trifoliatus: all are soap-nut. Vaccaria hispanica is another variety known as cowherb, cow cockle, cow basil, cow soapwort. All are sources for the soapberry used for cleaning the body. Details:

ii. Retha, Sapindas mukorossi, Sabuni- produced in Northern India.

iii. Kunkudu-kai (details): Sapindas trifoliatus: Arishtaka, Raktabeeja, Vishapushpak, South India Soap-nut, three-leaf soapberry, Sabuni, Soap-nut; Sapindas laurifolius is a synonym to S. trifoliatus – common to south India.

The soap-fruit pericarp is used as a good substitute of shampoo. It contains saponins, tri-terpenoids, fatty acids and flavonoids etc., It is a detergent and febrifuge. Also used in treatment of long-continued fevers.

iv. Shikakai (details): Acacia concinna, Acacia sinuata, Acacia hooperiana, Mimosa concinna, most well-known for the natural shampoo derived from its fruit. This is boiled in water for about half-an hour, to act as shampoo.

A2. Take half liter water after mouth wash. For that the body needs a clean drinking water. The best way is to collect water through muslin. Still during rainy days, water borne diseases float through water. So, clean water for drinking is a must and so prefer copper vessel to collect water. It cures the water.

Alternatively, the age-old technique is to use chilla-ginja. Chilla-ginja, Strychnos potato- rum, Tettamparal, Clearing-Nut Tree, Nirmali, Kataka; The seeds of the tree are commonly used in traditional system for purifying water in India and Myanmar. Seeds are used in the treatment of gonorrhea, leucorrhea, gastropathy, bronchitis, chronic diarrhea, dysentery, renal and vesicle calculi, diabetes, conjunctivitis, ulcers and other eye diseases.

A3. The next best is a cup of tea, with/without milk. Then after ½ hr. take a cup of tea. Or some prefer a cup of coffee and also coffee with/without chicory. Some people still prefer herbal drink either yarrow or Hypercom extracts, or neem leaf juice- that fall into the next level of treatments. If one refers to wiener's herbal, it is full of herbal teas. In case, tea is not preferred, go for fruit juices.

A4. The body needs stimulus in the morning as juices. Here, a glassful of fresh grape/orange juice is good. Amla and lemon and many Citrus plants are good as tonics.

i. All citrus fruits (details): are consumed with sugar/honey and many are pickled. They can be orange, lemon (Citrus limon), lime or Galgal or dabbakai, (Cochlospermum religiosum or can be Citrus pseudo- lemon). Another sour variety is gajanimma or Bijapuraka, known as jambira as a wild lemon slightly bigger than lemon, & smaller than sour fruits like Galgal and kimb.

   These are small evergreen trees, native to Asia. Jambira – are already discussed in Ganesh puja. Galgal is a medium sized wild or semi-wild fruit.

   Another is naranja- a sour juicy fruit, Bitter orange, Seville orange, or marmalade orange is probably a hybrid, long grown in India.

   A sweeter variety is battai probably Citrus aurantium. Some named Citrus limetta as Battai chettu- mostly its juice is given as a tonic during fevers and also drunk as a freshener, just like orange juice. Orange, or kamala and its brother kino are excellent juice yielding sweet – sour fruits.

   Citrus sinensis, also known as the sweet oranges, is a commonly cultivated family of oranges. All these plants are native to India

(Southeast Asia). All Citrus fruits and leaves contain limonene, with good odor & used for flavouring diluted buttermilk at every home.

ii. Angora, Vitis vinifera: Amritaphala,Svaduphala, Draksha, Amlavetasah, Gostani, Bush grape, three leaved wild vines; The sap of young branches possess activity like, Anti-oxidant, Anti-diabetic, Anti-microbial antiviral and Anti-carcinogenic effects and considered as a remedy for skin diseases, useful in thirst, heat of the body; leaves astringent, unripe fruits cure throat infection, & has malic & tartaric acids also. Its synonyms are Cissus trifoliate, Vitis trifoliate and Vitis carnosa.

Grape leaves are useful as paste for external application to rheumatism, pains, sprains, pillows stuffed with these dried leaves to cure catarrh and headache; leaf powder given in intermittent fevers; flowers prescribed medicine with honey for fevers also to prevent vomiting and even severe thirst; The herbs contain free radical scavengers like polyphenols, flavonoids etc. The herb is useful in capillary bleeding, in treating diabetes, edema, and inflammation from injury and radiation damage. Grapes are considered laxative, stomachic, diuretic, demulcent and cooling.

A5. Another set acid fruits are regu, mango, imli and also Garcinia etc., These acidic fruits/juices are also digestive or constipation eliminators and acidic in nature. Another set acid fruits are mango, imli and also Garcinia. These acidic fruits/juices are also digestive or constipation eliminators. Another sour fruit is mango, imli and also Garcinia. Thai imli is a sweet fruit – consumed as such, while Indian is sour-used in soups, chutneys etc.,

i. Ziziphus jujube, or regu, is well known medicinal uses- discussed in Ganesh puja. They are consumed raw and seed thrown out.

ii. Amla is another acid fruit, one of the three myrobalans, discussed already in spices. Amalaki, Emblica officinalis, Sriphala, Malacca tree, Phyllanthus emblica, Emblic Myrobalan, Dhatriphala, Usirikai, Indian Gooseberry; Amla means acidic; thus, fruits are rich in vitamin-C, coolant, diuretic, antioxidant, immune-modulatory, antipyretic; fruit used in jaundice; Its seeds used in asthma and bronchitis.

Its fruit acrid and is a natural source of citric acid and hence used for pickling. It is coolant, diuretic and laxative. The fermented fruits are used in jaundice. The flowers are used as cooling, refrigerant and aperients. Its root and bark are used as astringent. It is of two varieties, one for marmalade/pickling and another variety is only for raw consumption as it is sweetish sour.

iii. Amra, mamidi, Aam, Mangifera indica, commonly known as mango, is a fruit bearing plant. Mangoes are believed to have originated from India, northwestern Myanmar & Bangladesh.

Mango tree is rich in proteins, nutrients and vitamin C. Mango fruit is consumed and its unripe mango fruit is pickled. It is uterotonic (chut patta) and used to prevent bad omen. It is decorated for every good purpose. Mango tree leaves helps in keeping body energetic and prevent skin infection too.

iv. Imli, Siri Manu, Tamarindus indica, Tamarind is a tree. Its partially dried fruit is used to make chutney. People use tamarind for constipation, fever, gallbladder disorders, disorders affecting bile flow in the liver & is used traditionally for treating abdominal pain, diarrhea, and dysentery, wound healing, inflammation and also fever. It helps in digestion and also improves heart by reducing cholesterol levels. It also protects from liver malfunction.

v. Manna plant, Tamarix gallica, (syn T. troupe), French tamarisk, *Sirasamu*, Javnu, Jhadu, Pilli-chi, Tamarisk; it is found in abundance in North India, has laxative and anti-hemolytic. It has been used to staunch the flow of blood from wounds. It speeds up the healing process and a laxative too.

Its galls are astringent, given internally, in dysentery and diarrhea. Its manna is laxative, expectorant, detergent. Its galls contain @40% tannic acid.

vi. Amlavetasa, Garcinia pedunculata: Sohdanei, Bar thekera, is already discussed in spices. They are used to prepare juice, pickles and as acidulant in making sambar etc., curries. In the traditional Indian system of medicine, the Ayurveda and in various folk systems of medicine, the fruit rinds and leaves are used to treat various inflammatory ailments, rheumatic pain and bowel complaints. Kokum extracts are weight reducers also. Garcinia indica, a plant in the mangosteen family, commonly known as kokum, is with fruits with pharmaceutical uses.

More like Velaga, lasora, lasori, vaakkaya etc., are also acidic fruits and used as such or cooked or made chutney or pickled.

A6. Leaf therapy: Indian is lentil and fresh leaf-cooked soup, is consumed as such or with rice/bread. The green leafy vegetables which serve as body cleansers (laxatives) – some are as below.

Such treatments involve use of vegetables, spices and standard suggested herbs- of centuries old. Here, the plants are part of Indian food chain with healing powers/curative properties.

They supply vital minerals needed by the body and are also good demulcents. If one consumes Thota Kura (Amaranth leaf), palak (spinach), Gongora (Hibiscus sabdariffa), chukka Kura (sorrel leaves), Bachali (Basella alba, vine spinach), ponnaganti (water amaranth or copper dwarf leaf), etc., cooked leaves as soup, as one variety a day, where is the need for medicine. Here Malabar spinach or Ceylon bachali is insect resistant and rapidly grows at my home also and consumed like palak is also good.

i. Gongora is a sour leaf, digestive and is known as roselle plant (Hibiscus sabdariffa) grown for its edible leaves in India and in other countries like Fiji. Its brother known as Konda gogu, Hibiscus Cannabinus or karni-karamu-is less acidic. These leaves are used in south-central Indian cuisine. Gongora comes in two varieties, green stemmed leaf and red stemmed. Leaf is consumed as a tea, used as pulusu (soup), and even preserved as chutney for months. It is beneficial for high blood pressure too.

   Even its fruit petals – red in colour, when mixed with ripe capsicum makes excellent red chutney.-full of acids thereby digestive, laxative and it acts as demulcent also. Other chemicals in Gongora might be able to lower blood pressure, reduce levels of sugar and fats in the blood, reduce swelling, and acts as demulcent. Chukka-Kura (sorrel leaf) is another variety of sour leaf with more laxative properties and is used like Gongora.

ii. Thota Kura in Telugu-means Garden spinach or chulai in Hindi or Kuppacheera in Malayalam is scientifically known as the Amaranthus viridis (green Amaranthus). This is a green vegetable that is traditionally eaten as vegetable in South India. Still softer variety- is perugu totakura, and harder variety is koyya-Thota

Kura. Koyya-Thota Kura is hard to digest, yet widely used and they grow wild & also cultivated.

Malaysia uses Amaranthus spinosus as an expectorant and to relieve breathing in acute bronchitis, and also used as sudorific, febrifuge, galactagogue, and to treat menorrhagia. It may be different from the Indian varieties. In India all three variety Thota Kura exist both in red and green varieties.

iii. Spinach, also known as Spinacia oleracea- is a leafy green flowering plant native to central and western Asia. Its leaves are a common edible vegetable consumed after cooking or either fresh or after storage by canning or freezing. Spinach is of the amaranth family grown widely at homes and consumed.

iv. Basella alba or Malabar spinach or Ceylon bachali is an edible perennial vine in the family Basellaceae. It is widely used as a leaf vegetable- even grown at my home.

v. Bachali, Basella alba, Indian traditional is of green and red varieties and both are creepers. Basella alba is an edible perennial vine in the family Basellaceae. It is widely used as a leaf vegetable, grown at home.

vi. Ponnaganti- kura, Alternanthera sessilis/Sessile Joy weed/Dwarf Copperleaf- is a flowering plant known by several common names, Malabar spinach. It is variously known as matikaduri in Assamese, ponnanganni, ponnaganti aku, honnagone, and mukunuwenna. It is also known as Matsyaakshi, Ponnonkanni keerai, Ponnanganni, Mukunuwenna, Gudari Saag, and as Water Amaranth.

vii. Eclipta prostrata, commonly known as false daisy, Gunta kalagaraku/Gunta galagara-aku, Karisalankanni, and bhringraj, is a species of plant. This potent formulation of bhringraj is extremely effective in increasing appetite, aiding in digestion, and improving body metabolism. Other benefits of bhringraj oil · May promote relaxation and sleep · May help prevent urinary tract infections. It also helps in liver detoxification, hair loss, grey hair & helps in hair re-growth. The best way to use bhringraj is making hair oil with it as it cools brain too. Bhringraj has numerous health benefits like offering relief from respiratory disorders & relieving pain. Chemically similar to the hormone estrogen and hence emmenagogue.

Still, there is broccoli, cabbage-green and red varieties-leafy vegetables available as substitutes to the above list. Here even moor Konda leaf, mulaga leaf, castor oil leaf or even punarnava leaves are consumed once a while along with some lentil- well cooked. If one uses one of the above leaves once in three days, their health problems may minimize in to-to.

viii.   Alfa-alfa, Medicago sativa; it is a perennial plant. Its leaf consumption reduces sensitivity to pollens and its consumption also lowers cholesterol, cures Kidney troubles; but seeds toxic; traditionally alfalfa is used as antioxidant, anti-diabetic agent & relieve kidneys & menopause symptoms. Alfalfa is high in plant compounds called Phyto-estrogens, which are

A7. Constipation removers; Fruits and raw vegetables Salads: Tomato, Solanum Lycopersicon- is another acidic vegetable and used for chutney, also as soup & sauce, and also taste maker as salad. Since salad issue came up, Radish, carrot, Kheera, onion both bulb and shoots, beet root, broccoli, alfa-alfa etc., serve as salads. In Northern parts, kakri is a tasty seasonal vegetable for raw consumption during lunch and dinners. Here steamed cabbage leaves, muli, gajar, beet root, etc.

A8. Fruits: Banana, papaya, mango, anar, panasa, sapota, Seetha-phal, ram phal etc. Are widely available for consumption.

3b. Body needs Energy through Cereals

Whether rice or bread, it needs one or more cereals to make a meal. Here, wheat, rice, tur dal, chick-pea (chana dal), green gram, white beans (bobbarlu), black sesame, Kulatha (ulavalu), ragi, black gram (minumulu)} – named as nine cereals for routine food.

Another common vegetable cum medicine belongs to Alliums group (Onion, Allium cepa: Pyaz, Garden onion, Palandu; Garlic, Allium sativum, (bulb/its clove); Lasson, Welsh onion, Allium fistulosum: Japanese bunching onion). Allium as a spice is already discussed. After food pan with calcium, one need to apply katha as it reduces calcium caused sores on tongue. Khadira, Acacia catechu, Khair, Katha- are different names for this plant. Acacia is used like an astringent. Used in stomach problems like diarrhea, dysentery, colitis and also gastric cancer. It is used as a mouth wash and used for treating mouth, gum and throat problems. The extract is also used for treating hemorrhages and blood pressure also. It contains many phenolic compounds like 4- hydroxybenzoic acid, kaempferol, quercetin, 3,4',7-trihydroxyl-3',5- dimethoxy-flavone, catechin, epicatechin, afzelechin, epi-afzelechin, mesquitol, phenol, catechin, catechuic acid, phloroglucinol, quercetin, gum, and minerals. Its extract is called katha, applied on pan to act as a coolant for calcium (single calcium on betel leaf causes sores on tongue) and hence a soothing mineral carrier. I grow pan (Naga Valli) creeper at home and consume it gulkand, Elachi and lavang, betelnut supari, whenever digestive need arises.

3.c. Fire Sterilization and Vegetable Therapy

The next level of therapy is by using fire or using spices/herbs/ vegetables- through cooking. Hence can be called home remedies as every kitchen is a health gainer. This is the difference between good old days and the present-day- as every family needs a physician now even for minor ailment because even basic herbs are not grown. Is it a progress or downfall- one has to judge.

The next step is tinkering with human system using food. Such treatments involve use of vegetables, spices and standard suggested herbs- of centuries old. Here, the vegetable plants are part of Indian food chain with healing powers/curative properties.

They supply vital minerals needed by the body and are also good demulcents. If one consumes cooked leaves one variety a day, where is the need for medicine. Here Malabar spinach or Ceylon bachali is insect resistant and rapidly grows at home and consumed like palak is also good.

Even for rapidly transmitting diseases, another vegetable like patola (also known as chedu-potla – exclusively used as medicine). But, its brothers- like, birakai (ridged guard, tori), potlakai (snake guard, chic inga), & potals- also have insect and bacterial resistant properties, yet serve as vegetables.

In fact, the ripened seeds of birakai (Ridged guard) are used as an external application by boiling them in oil for all sours and hardened itch. Here anapa (Lauaki), gummadi – sweet (meetha – kaddu, Cucurbita pepo) or gummadi— sour or budida-gummadi (petha, Benincasa hispida), panasa (jackfruit), kheera (cucumber) etc., are also good. Tribal's use dried ripened Lauaki empty shells like thermos flask to carry water!

Another well-known vegetable is vankaya that belong to the family of brihati – or buri Hathi or Bir Hathi which is a well-known medicinal plant and vankaya leaves (vartaki, baingan, Solanum melongena), also look similar to brihati leaves and vartaki most useful vegetable, while others are good medicines.

Another important vegetable is teepi gummadi – a natural zinc supplier or budida-gummadi – a natural weight enhancer. Even tori, maximum produced in North India, also called neti birakai is also not prone to insects.

Story: Thus, in order to elaborate it, there is a story on vegetables as mentioned here. All vegetables went to tomato to select a suitable companion for it. Then tomato dribbled over all vegetables and settled near palandu (onion). Then many of the vegetables became jealous and went to bhindi (okra) to protest against their being neglected. Then bhindi questioned tomato- how it rated palandu to be superior to all. Then tomato blushed a while, with its cheeks developing deep red color-then replied.

You bhindi, if you are not used in prime time & cut late, you become hard and unfit for consumption too. The next, you are not as stable as petha which hangs for months to the ceiling and cures even bad omen for a new house. It also with sugar become halwa or as a stable sweet- called petha for regular consumption.

Neither you are comparable to the king of vegetables vartaki, which mixes with all vegetables including meat preparations with ease. You are not as nutritional as beans. Further, you are not as worm resistant as potlakai (Snake guard or chic inga), Birakai, potal & teepi gummadi. Here, kakara (karela) or mulaga or munaga (drumstick),-all are vegetables and also selective medicines.

Can you compare yourself with Lauaki (kaddu) which help in weight reduction and thus help the heart? Since the talk on heart has come, can you compare yourself to Dondakaya, Ivy Gourd or tindora- which serve as cardiotonic? Nakka-dosakai (khatta kheera) is another is age-old local variety of AP. It is rarely attacked by insects and used as raw with spice & salt or it is even pickled (avakaya). You are not even useful as kheera (cucumber), carrot, tomato, alfalfa, cabbage, onion etc. that serve as salads.

Look at panasa, an insect resistant and most useful vegetable. After taking all vital fruit lobes with seeds from jackfruit, the soft strands inside the fruit are fried in oil and served as evening snack-- good for diabetics. Here, mango, pomegranate or boppai (papaya) also serve as vegetables and fruits. Plus, there are many fruits like Ber (ziziphus) as immune-modulator or neredu (Jambul) as diabetes cure, orange, chiku (sapota)- a stomach cleaner, banana- an antacid, etc., good regular use fruits and Anas a (pineapple)-as laxative, vit. A rich & so on,- which are seasonal.

Now, look at palandu (onion) as it is a poor man's vegetable cum bactericide, even serves as vegetable and salad for eating with rice or roti or bread along with hari-mirch (green chili) & salt – that too raw! It is again palandu (onion) which is crushed and applied as poultice on insect bites or even scorpion bites. It grows in deep winter when many vegetables fail to grow. Further, onion & its shoots are consumed raw as salad. It is again palandu (onion) that helps eyes when tear gas shell bursts. It is also a good staple food for months together like potatoes and other rhizomes. Yet, your okra, still beneficial as you clean the entire gastrointestinal tract.

Before tomato could extend further discussion, the chef arrived and took onion and cut to pieces and he put it into frying pan with oil and then cut tomato and put into it. Laughingly tomato says it is again palandu which stayed ahead of me in cooking also. Thus, after tomato's end, all vegetables started looking at each other, waiting for the chef's hand to fall- as they are not sure of their turn!

This is a story about routinely consumed vegetables for several generations- with no side effects. Today also, when a person falls sick, the patient is advised to shun meat or animal foods and consume cooked vegetables with spices.

3.d: Reducing (impact of) diseases: Some vegetables & fruits help the human system in reducing impact of the following diseases as below:

High blood pressure: apple, lemon, garlic, red rice, use less oil in foods and less salt content or use Sindhava salt.

Congestion of lungs: tulasi, pudina,

Intoxication: khajjur

Gall stones: Take papaya along with a glassful of boiled and concentrated water (reduced to $1/5^{th}$ level) for three months.

Hyper-acidity: Napata, mango, arhar dal, ground nut, gummadi-teepi seeds, vegetable salads, honey, milk, Bael fruit, or Bael leaf consumption as such or as extract.

Whooping cough: garlic, ginger dried powder, muli (radish), bad-am, reduces its on set, but drastic medicine if struck.

Diabetes- reducing-: amla, mango leaf, karela (kakara), green gram (pesalu), menthe (menthulu), kaddu (Lauaki), soyabean nutria, tomato, chana dal, urad dal, ground nut.

Urinary troubles: beet root, danimma, banana, grapes, amla, kaddu (anapakai), khira (dosa kai), methi leaf, green leaf, onion, mango leaf juice.

Heart disease: apple, grapes, danimma, amla, orange, garlic, onion, wheat, arhar dal.

Muscle pain: Mustard oil or seed paste, Ravi stem paste.

Obesity: lemon, lime, cabbage, tomato, ground nut, honey.

Kidney diseases: fruits like banana, grapes, dates, apple, anar.

Lumbago: lime, lemon, garlic.

Liver activation: grapes, sugarcane juice, jambool (neredu fruit or leaf/stem/bark ext.), mango, tomato, danimma, coconut.

Jaundice: lemon, lime, mango, danimma, beet root, ginger, muli (radish) ext., butter milk.

Intestinal disorders: banana, butter milk, dates, papaya.

Insomnia: vegetable soup, kaddu (anapa), curd, butter milk, avoid oily foods at night.

Laxatives: Panasa (jack fruit), pineapple fruit, Cassia leaves, drumstick leaves as rasam, bhindi (okra)- as demulcent, leafy vegetables, and fruits.

Prevention of diarrhea: banana, curd.

3.e: Health Tips

Thus, the impact of diseases can be brought down with simple means. If such simple measures do not work, better to consult a physician or I present below one such easy viable disease resistant tonic which also is said to cure in its onset and is as under.

i. The most delicious choice is banana- best source for vitamins a, b, c and e, along with potassium.

    Another example is jam-Bira (Atalantia malabarica or Adivi nimma) as its fruit – used like lemon and leaf oil or fruit peel oil- serve for external application in rheumatism and paralysis.

ii. All neuro problems, including male infertility can be resolved with betel leaf-applied with honey & sankh- bhasma 300 mg It is consumed early morning empty stomach. Later no tea or coffee or chocolate is to be taken that day. But one can consume milk with sugar and haldi everyday; such extreme treatments are not in use now.

iii. iii. These are some old theories and no one scientifically verified, but accepted by tradition. There are some forbidden – A combination like consumption of egg and potlakai (chic inga) is termed to be poisonous.

iv. Also pregnant mother should not consume boppai (pepita, or papaya, Ficus carica) as it can cause abortion in early stages.

v. v. There is another problem- like eating fish and milk or its preparations together which can cause allergy or psoriasis.

vi. Further, if one consumes brinjal, it also aggravates itch. If one avoids non-vegetarian products like milk, egg and meat, half the health problems, including mental problems can get reduced.

vii. vii. Similarly, strengthening womb walls is increased by consumption of jammi flowers with sugar.

How far these are more useful or they are only superstitions-I don't know.

viii. A good vegetable is Cucurbit-a pepo,-it being worm expeller besides its seeds rich in zinc, magnesium, selenium, phosphorus and even iron.

ix. ix. Even simple cabbage has Sulphur, chlorine, iodine and iron in it. Almonds are rich in fatty acids, magnesium, iron, phosphorus, copper, and even potassium- making it a good enzymatic nut.

x. x. An apple a day keeps doctor away. Even a simple vegetable like drumstick or even its plant leaves are good laxatives. Kakara is used as wormicide, anti-diabetic and stomach curative.

3.f. Garlic as Medicine

I avoided garlic in regular food as my grandmother did so. For bringing down cholesterol levels in blood, I was suggested to take garlic as a medicine. But, as a scientist, I tested it by consuming three lobes of garlic like a capsule and took water early morning. Within three minutes it entered blood and burnt all – along the path of blood for five minutes and subsided. Allicin is a powerful medicine (like an antibiotic), if taken alone. But, it is effective,- provided you are not a regular consumer of garlic in food! After two months, what I find is that digestion improved and cholesterol levels came down.

3.g: The Food Additives

Spices are used all over the world since ages as food additives and hence their efficacy/usefulness is beyond doubt. Their consumption changes from region to region and also differ from continent to continent.

Many spices of regular use- attack gram positive and gram-negative bacilli and thus secretly protecting us. The publications on spices amply support this contention. In Indian peninsula, there are @fifty in number, constitute back bone for survival by using them as taste makers. One needs to add spices as bacilli grow faster in warm climates. Their list is given later chapters along with spicy herbs.

3.h: Stomach Problems

some specific treatments are needed for the diseases which begin with stomach associated problems (udara-roga). Agnimandya (indigestion) or Jala, Vayu dosha- (indigestion), or distension of abdomen, or vilambaca (constipation),- thus all create problems due to the hypoacidity.

A. The patient is the judge in his treatment and is done with the use of honey 5 gm. with water early morning.

B. Indigestion (agnimandya) is simply cured with lemon juice and salt thrice daily or in rasam preparations or both. Then select spice as below:

C. Haldi and jeera- Jeera soup aids to clear indigestion and stimulate the production of enzymes-thereby treating acne, anemia, cough and cold.

D. Black pepper-. Black pepper soup eases digestion, cough and stimulates the stomach, It prevent mental depression, cancer, and Improves skin. It also improves bioavailability of many drugs in the body.

E. Hingu- The gum resin of Ferula species, known as hingu-is laxative, anti-spasmodic, carminative, expectorant & cures hysteria, some nervous conditions, sedative and cures whooping cough. It is also useful in the treatment of infantile pneumonia and flatulent colic. Hing is teratogenic too for worms and bacilli inside our body, while its effects are minimal for us. At the time of conception, even women are advised to skip this drug, Hing.

F. Dhania- boiled for ten minutes- boiled for ten minutes. The soup is helpful in loss of appetite, excessive thirst, & treats bacilli infections.

G. Ginger as soup (one spice at a time in soup only) beneficial. boiled for ten minutes. It is viswabheshaja- cures all evils.

H. Western way is the starter soup of vegetables with salt & pepper. Indian vegetable soup (rasam, pulusu or sambar) is consumed with rice or idly. It contains imli most digestive along with spices, salt, jiggery.

I. with laxative effects is mulaga-leaf containing rasam. It empties stomach in about two hours and person is normal same day much better than senna. So, rasam or sambar (spice and salt rich cousins) provides salts in artificial way. But, Sambhar Lake of Rajasthan provides vital salts to many cattle and thus the word sambar is probably evolved from here.

J. Taking vitamin C at least 1/2 gm per day – is said to have been recommended by the Nobel laureate Linus Pauling for a better health. So, instead the tablet, one can consume amla or mango pickle or chywanprash, or amla candy, amla juice or even its chutney. The next best choice is oranges-all varieties- as such or as fruit juice or squash. In the Indian tradition vitamin C or its equivalent is consumed routinely as a tasty food – instead a tablet.

Thus, through the regular food, the healing process can be tinkered.

3.i: Avoid oily foods and high salt diet, for a qualitative sleep. Take curd and rice- best menu for a good sleep. But the sleeplessness is a most common problem that exists with most humans since their birth.

For example, a person is in deep forest and it is infested with wolves, tigers, and snakes etc.,-so, out of fear, he cannot afford to sleep. But, coming to the present-day life, insomnia or sleeplessness poses a basic problem. Animals sleep at night or sometimes yell, which means some stranger, entered the area or snake nearby or there is an anticipated earth quake.

In humans, the desires shadow during the sleep time. Even during Ramayana days, the king Dashrath was sleepless because he granted two boons to his wife Kaikeye. At the end of Mahabharat war, Ashwatthama (Drona's son), killed upa-Pandeva-s in sleep & proposed a new definition for sleeplessness by adding more points for it. He said "the people who possess excess wealth or one whose wealth is stolen or one who is fond of lust, or angry/revengeful groups that develop anguish – are likely to be sleepless. My doctor friend advised me in dinner, take food like a pauper, without oil and with salads.

3.j: Animal Foods and Bacilli

The bacilli need foods of animal origin like meat or egg or milk – means food of animal origin for faster growth-inside the body. There are auto immune diseases that can affect our health.

In such cases ayurveda offers simple solution-i.e., one step stoppage of all (Vegan policy)- avoiding such foods of animal origin, including milk & curd! This does not mean all diseases can be tackled with vegetables and spices only. Depending upon severity, more drastic measures needed to tackle these troubles later.

Though, the life expectancy had goneup from 55 years to 69 years, at what cost? At the cost of large consumption of modern medicines. The negative effects of synthetic medicines is also high.

The point noteworthy is that if meat consumers do not exist, there will be more animals can eliminate total available vegetation. Then, so called vegan group will be left with no grass or vegetable for survival. Hence, the age-old rulers used hunting to eliminate excess animals.

In Australia helicopter strafed bullets kill many kangaroos so that greenery is retained in the region. But a man living near poles or in snow clad regions or entrapped persons at sea, have to bank on fish or meat products for survival. India is blessed with jungles – rich in flora & fauna.

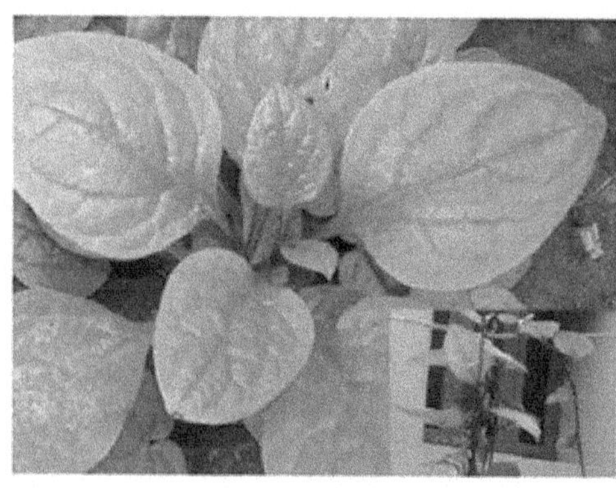

Bacchali creeper

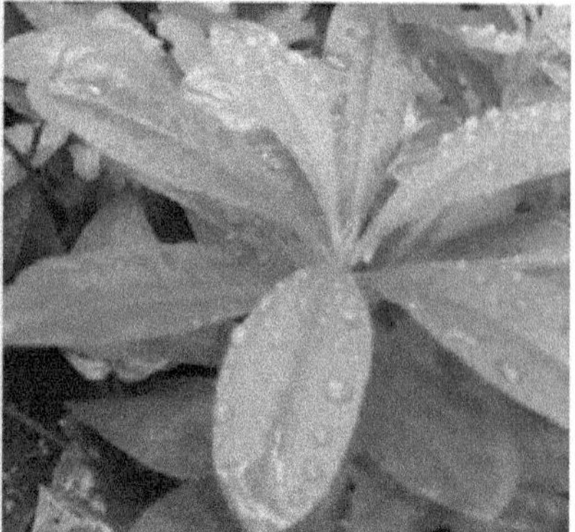

Ceylon bacchali shrub

Some home- grown plants

Finally the saying is- "only eat food for living, lest it can eat your health and wealth too."

4. Chemistry

Role of chemistry: In general, every fact-finding mission (sat or truth) cannot work without chemistry – as- most body reactions are chemical in nature or in other words, the human/animal body or even a tree are true chemical factories. Here, each specie produces compounds that are characteristic to its genes.

Thus, all species of Curcuma contains curcumin. But the highest concentration of it is in Curcuma longa (haldi). It is extractable with alcohol or acetone and when it is purified & analyzed by HPLC, it contains 67% keto and 33% enol form (my unpublished results). Similarly, every human or every animal express his/its own character physically or biologically or chemically or genetically.

It is the plant chemical analysis that gave compounds like, quercetin, rutin, vasicine, 67 piperine, atropine, reserpine, strychnine, etc.. Similarly, several protein hormones like insulin, FSH, LH, TSH etc., were isolated and analyzed-in protein chemistry. Using the modern spectral analysis, any chemical constituent present in the tonic or tablet (goli) can be deciphered.

The chemistry helps in obtaining the basic drug from non-conventional sources-including synthetic means also. Further, it also helps in the discovery of new related drugs. Here, crude petroleum is analyzed to provide vital intermediates for medicines at cheapest cost- again chemistry.

Even ayurveda used such natural drugs as concentrated vati in medicine – after compounding with other exepients like guduchi or ashwagandha satwa, aloe juice or tamarind seed powder etc., polymers used.

Vati or goli means a concentrated pill. Here, one can locate an alternative source of drug- in the substitution of a plant product- to generate similar effect. There are large numbers of herbs in Charak Samhita preparations and absence of vital drug, rendering ayurvedic drug ineffective too.

But, addition of use me too type drugs, bio-enhancers, color, flavor, taste makers & stabilizers- led to the bulging of every type of medicinal system & a common problem with modern drugs also.

Hence, the modern thinking of herbal medicine – by using herbs in a holistic way is developed to bypass ayurveda. But, in herbal medicine also, (like modern drugs) some inbuilt toxicity that exist in some herbs. Hence, compounding is necessary. Thus, use medicine with care and abandon it at the earliest after recovery.

4.ii. What is pH

So,what is pH and how it is evolved? It is the hydrogen ion concentration in the fluid-expressed as negative logarithm to the base ten. Generally, water dissociates as below.

$$2H_2O \rightleftharpoons H_3O^+ + OH^-$$

It means water has some reversible dissociation constant and at the equilibrium, the ion strength is measurable using electrodes. Thus, water is known to be at pH 7 (H^+ ion concentration is $= 1X10^{-7}$). If acidic- there is more hydrogen ion concentration and hence its pH will be less than 7. Similarly, if alkaline, the pH will be hence more than 7.

Thus, Sulphuric acid has pH1, vinegar has pH2 and lemon juice is in between 1 and 3pH. Milk has 6.5 to 6.8 pH and a healthy water lake has 6.5 pH. Similarly, sea water has pH 8, ammonia pH 11 and soap water has pH 12.

Then what about the blood, it is 7.4 pH. Thus, the word Ph had simplified the understanding of acids and bases. Coming to the human body, it has a complex mechanism to create different pH zones within the body- like stomach acidic and intestines alkaline etc., the blood proteins are the most important buffers in the body and they try to eliminate every drug through metabolism- again through blood. Thus, proteins also regulate the pH as required at the site of action in the body-which involve inorganic metal-chemistry (more treatment details in the next chapter).

4.iii. Hemoglobin and Chlorophyll

The porphin structure in chlorophyll- absorbs carbon dioxide (along with sunlight) and water through roots- and releases oxygen into the air in a regular way (photo-synthesis). Here, formaldehyde polymerizes to sugars and polymers. Some plants producing beans have nitrogen fixing capability to prepare amino acids & so on.

$$CO2 + H2O \rightarrow HCO3H + h\surd \text{ (sun light)--- } \rightarrow 2\ HCHO + O2$$

In a human body too, the blood contains another heme structure to absorb oxygen from air during respiration and exhale carbon dioxide. The iron-known as heme is linked to blood proteins-known as globulins- making it red hemoglobin. Thus, both chlorophyll and hemoglobin-have capabilities to absorb the desired molecule through air using multivalent metal ions.

It is chlorophyll that needs UV light for photosynthesis and the body uses UV light to break phytosterols. In both places inorganic ions flip their valence state.

It is the same blood that brings back Fe^{2+} to the lungs whereby the blood is recharged with oxygen in lungs to convert it to Fe^{3+}- it means a switch-over of oxidation states of iron ion.

Conspicuously, Indian Vada with a hole in the center is offered to elders on their death anniversary of parents-probably like expressing thanks for providing an excellent Heme structure.

Vada also depicts structure of a black hole (which also looks similar-where all fluffy stars move around it). Probably, all departed souls as atoms merge into the ultimate there.

There are many chemical reactions like oxidation & reduction; hydrolysis, esterification, even protein synthesis, etc.,- in the body and for all such activities, oxygen is supplied through the conversion of Fe^{3+} to Fe^{2+} or ATP or NADH or NADPH.

4.iv. Trouble Shooting

In the body every stress or strain, injury or pain – all have some chemical release like arachidonic acid/adrenaline/epinephrine/endorphins etc. Addition of herb or drug is a chemical process and its elimination is also a systematic chemical process. Here, the metal ions- known as dhatu provide help by holding allergens or forming complexes to eliminate them.

Ama: It is ama (acid) accumulation in joints that cause severe pain due to the release of acids. In order to cure it, pumping glucosamine orally along with other active components-as medicine is also done, yet bacilli hide and overcome total elimination, needing more drastic herbs.

Prostaglandins: Pain. Stress releases the Arachidonic acid- is rapidly dissipated into prostaglandins or leukotrienes. But every chemical process consumes energy causing weakness in the body- due to the disease.

When a person is given an injection of H^3-prostaglandin on one hand, it was not locatable on the other hand even if blood is drawn simultaneously (old reports of Scientific American).

But when an arthritis/inflammation struck animals were observed, there are higher prostaglandin E levels (unpublished reports) in blood. It means pain/stress is nearly proportional to prostaglandin E levels in the body.

4.v. Chemicals as Medicine

In my childhood apc (adenine, pethidine, caffeine) tablet was the medicine. Later came para-acetamol and so on. Now Sulphonyl urea derivatives have the capacity to generate hypoglycemic action and ethylene diamine tetra acetic acid or amides- commonly known as aminophylline is capable to reducing asthmatic tendencies.

Para-acetamido – phenol, aspirin or morphine serve as analgesics and anti-pyritic. Thus, chemicals are excellent regulators of health-as sugar substitutes, anti-pyretic, anti-biotics, analgesics, anti-diabetics, anti-inflammatory drugs etc. It is a known fact that any molecule's hypoglycemic capacity can be estimated by Keir's triangle through a formula and this led to create many new sugar substitutes- thanks to the petroleum products!

Ayurveda uses the cow urine it destroys glycoside bonds attached to the drug and its concentration increases with urine treatment (confirmed by Japanese research papers).

So, the ayurvedic techniques like soaking herbs in cow urine for about a week or more and extract the product with alcohol. Even-use as such by grinding plant herb-after a brief wash and drying. They use that powder with improved potency as drug. Even for a sluggish liver, ornithine tablets are compounded to increase activity in liver whereas ayurvedics use curry leaf (Muraya koengii) for stimulating liver. So, such similarities in use of herbs and medicines always exist.

4. vi. Herbs as Medicine

Now the question arises such as-is there any useful ayurvedic herb at present? In the independent India, by CSIR (Sir R.N. Chopra et.al.) consolidated the information on medicinal herbs as a Glossary of medicinal plants. But there is no mention of diabetes in the entire list.

It means, it is not a problematic disease in India. If the data of herbal trade of 2008 looked into, there are about two hundred plant species – that are either exported or imported in tons throughout the world (NPMB reports).

Even, the European commission in- @1994 made a list of 130 useful plants- despite of their strong hold on synthetic as well as biologically prepared medicines.

4.vii. Organic Classification of Herbs

Here the ayurvedic plant drugs can be comfortably divided based upon modern chemistry, as below: How the medicinal herbs have a capacity to tackle or cure some diseases and what do they contain? Here, the modern chemistry is useful in segregation of herbs based upon the compounds present in them, for example;

A. Phenolic compounds: These compounds form a group called tikta in ayurveda, Picrorrhiza   kurroa roots (katuki, katuka-rohini), Curcuma longa, Zingiber officinale, and other species, Andrographis paniculata folium (chiraita, kirata tikta), Swertia chirata (chiraita), Matricaria chamomilla, Gossypium herbaceum- or simple eugenol-based cloves, Ocimum sanctum herba, Psidium guajava, Rheum emodi, Ageratum conyzoides, Cinnamomum tamala etc.,

B. Gallic acid rich: pashanbhed (Bergenia ligulata), Cicca acida (syn Phyllanthus distichus),- in other words- all patharchur- herbs, plus Terminalia chebula or Terminalia belerica etc.,

C. Benzoic acid based: bamboo manna, Celastrus paniculatus, Inula helenium, etc.,

D. Organic acids based: Tamarindus indica fructus, Tamarix gallica, Citrus fruits or lemon and lime containing, Crataegus oxycantha fruits, Crescentia cujeti (bilayeti bel), fruit rind of Garcinia, amla fruit, Kalanchoe pinnata (asthibhaksha), Lycopersicon esculentum (tomato), Feronia acidissima (velaga) fruit, fruit of Mangifera indica, even the seeds of Punica granatum (anar-dana) etc., used.

E. Quercetin or rutin based: Capparis spinosa. Fagopyrum esculentum, Lycopersicon esculentum (tomato), Ruta graveolens, Sambucus nigra, Tephrosia purpurea, Viola odorata, Eucalyptus species. Euphorbia hirta/E. pulilifera, Mimosa pudica etc.,

F. Anthraquinone/naphtho-quinone/benzoquinone based: Rheum emodi, Cassia fistula, Aloe vera, Morinda citrifolia roots (togaru), Morinda umbellate (shiranji), Plumbago zeylanica (chitrak), Embelia ribes (vidanga), Lawsonia inermis (mehndi) etc., drugs.

G. Organic Sulphur based: Ferula narthex (asafetida), Brassica nigra (mustard), Allium cepa and Allium sativum, jangly pyaz etc.,

H. Spices: They are the safest medicines for thousands of years and even known for their bactericidal actions. Here, piperine containing piper species like white, black and long peppers are the most common spices. They are rich in aroma and phenolics.

I. Asparagine based: Abroma Augusta; Abutilon indicum, Asparagus officinalis, Hamulus lupulus, Platanus orientalis etc.,

J. j. Alkaloids: Another biggest and potent medicinal group of alkaloids. It can be quinine based like Cinchona officinalis used for malaria; serpentine alkaloids like Rauwolfia serpentina- for high blood pressure; Vasicine based bronchodilators like Adhatoda vasica and Peganum harmala; Opium alkaloids as pacifiers from Papaver somniferum; Conessine alkaloids anti–amoebic drugs from Hollarrhena antidysenterica; Piper alkaloids from Piper species for bactericidal action, given in TB to enhance potency of other drugs;

K. Berberine based like Berberis aristata and other species as anti-diarrheal; Atropa (Hyoscine) alkaloids from Atropa and Datura species for eye sterilization or dilation; Strychnine, brucine and bucatini containing alkaloids are known from Strychnos and Taxus species bactericidal; Ergot alkaloids produced through fungi; Even the hallucinogens are also based on lysergic acid derivatives isolated from hemp (Cannabis sativa).

L. Colchicine is an alkaloid available from Iphigenia indica, Colchicum autumnale or species of Colchicum, Gloriosa superba-or Gloriosa species. Colchicine levels in Gloriosa superba corms have been reported to the level of around 0.9%.- mostly used for gout and to kill warts in the body.

M. Antitumor drugs: Catechin in green tea, leafy vegetables of Brassica, Raphanus sativus, Combretum caffrum, Dysoxylum binectariferum, Papaver somniferum, Papaver somniferum, Maclura pomifera, Dereeis Malaccensis, vinca rosea or Catharanthus roseus, Taxus buccata or T. brevifolia,

Podophyllum peltatum,- are known plants for anti-tumor activity.

N. Ephedrine based: Ma Huang (ephedra) or Pinellia ternata is used in Chinese medicine. Ephedra species or Sida cordifolia used Indian medicine for similar effects. A sea grape (Coccoloba uvifera) is known to be used in America and the Caribbean, used to treat vomiting, bronchitis, & also hay fever etc.,

O. Ginseng/Pseudo-ginseng: Aralia cachemerica; Panax Ginseng and related species – used as tonic and so on. The above mentioned are a spec in the ocean of natural herbs. Even sea foods, animal foods, sea herbs, including sea salt find use as daily medicines.

Thus, the modern chemistry provides a person to substitute an active herb with another. What about inorganic metals?

Do they have some effects on our living?

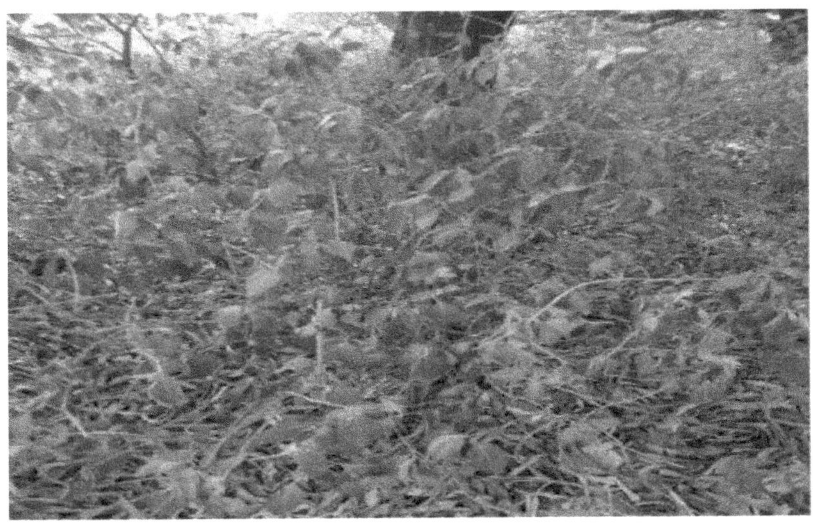

Ashwagandha

5. Metals/Minerals as Medicines

Do metals have a curing capacity? – One must say-Yes, it is possible. For example, the sodium/potassium (Na/K) ratios that determine the blood pressure and it is Cu/Mg ratios determine actions at the nerve junctions. Some sex stimulants can be tin or zinc or some other metal ions. Similarly, the absence of calcium ion means no insulin release at cellular levels. There are many metal ions that help in the body actions. Can we ignore iron presence in hemoglobin in blood? The problematic gall-bladder/kidney stones are also some inorganic – oxalates.

Further, there are a number of acid-base reactions, oxidative reactions, aldehyde- amino reactions, in which the metal ions serve as mediators – a novel example is zinc which catalyses more than three hundred enzymes in the body. Here, I find that some metallic complexes with herbs are used as strong medicines – specific to a disease. What are such metallic ions and what are such diseases?- many polyvalent metal ions do that trick.

Here, each metal ion in water is an alkali and alkaloids (alkali like) are well known for their prominent pharma-cological activities. Most of the metal ions enter the body through food chain. These are further supplemented as herbs or tablets or capsules or syrups or even as herbal tea. So, what are such inorganic ions?

Sapta dhatu: To mention a few,- gold, silver, copper, zinc, magnesium, manganese, selenium, chromium- besides daily needs of sodium, potassium, iron, and calcium – are needed. Here non-metallic ions like chlorides, phosphates, iodine or iodides and sulphur or sulphates- are also needed by the body in furthering some reactions. There is a notion that manganese reduces mental activity and silver sharpens the mental activity. Further gold or/and colored stones filter bad omens. These are suggested to be seven dhatus in the body and all dhatus carry metal ions for action. Thus, the body needs even- lead, aluminum, tin, cobalt, arsenic and even mercury- depending upon the situation. The physician is the best judge in suggesting the combinations.

5.i. Shilajit, the Rocky Asphalt

Coming to shilajit, a rocky asphalt – a bituminous substance-containing more than 50% fulvic acid in it along with many minerals. It is considered as 'sarva- roga-nivarini' (cures all diseases). It has some gold and silver salts in it and some silajit-s are reported to have more than 85 elements in it. The real shilajit collected below the shallow slopes of mountains with vital metallic ions is good and powerful.

However, there are several duplicates available in the market, using metal scrap boiled with cow and goat urines or a metal admixture burnt with cow dung. There are some of the standard procedures adopted by ayurvedic practitioners – to improve metallic contents in the collected shilajit. But some quarks use the same very techniques to supply duplicated materials. Thus comes the adulteration. This had brought bad name to ayurvedics too.

Some ayurvedic preparations include addition of metal ash-called bhasma. A novel example is that of Lord Shiva – known as Bhasma-anga-ragaya (who always wears bhasma). Now one uses talcum powder which is also a modern bhasma.

5.ii. Sambhar Lake

In Rajasthan-there exists a Salt Lake called Sāmbhar. The lake receives water from five rivers: Medtha, Samaod, Mantha,

Rupangarh, Khari, and Khandela. Lake has 5700 square km catchment area. It provides good mineral nutrition to many animals. It also serves many people with basic mineral needs in summer.

Even rice boiled water with salt is also given as a summer drink in student hostels of some parts of India (-called ganji and if preserved in pot for days together called tarwani which is my childhood energy drink). Soup, sambar and rasam- the Indian cousine are salt and spice rich fluids.

5.iii. Metal Ion Eliminations

Here, (P.B. chakrawarti), the stability of metal complexes vis-à-vis cephalosporins attracted my attention. The stability of metal complexes is in the following order $Cu^{2+} > Zn^{2+} > Co^{2+} > Ni^{2+} > Cd^{2+} > Mg^{2+} > Mn^{2+}$. Thus, if zinc and magnesium supplements are given, the detoxification in the body can be done. The pumpkin is recommended for regular use as wormicide and tonic as it and its seeds are rich in zinc complexes. The copper, if present in larger amount acts as a poison in the body- though its capacity to kill some bacilli is known. E every rishi or sanyasi used to carry water in copper vessels in good old days. Even today one can see fresh Ganga waters getting sealed in a copper vessel in Hardwar and I also carried two such vessels to home. Here copper sulphate is also used an important

medicine-marketed as supradyn. In ayurveda use of boiled water, concentrated to

levels- is cooled and used as a body cleaner because it is a rich source of magnesium.

Temples and metals: A number of metals are layered below deity or below dhwaja stamba (pillar) and said to absorb bad omens. The worn articles like pancha loha kada (five metal hand/foot bracelets), and sapta dhatu rings (seven metal rings) also are available near temples along with copper, brass and bronze articles. Brass (ittadi) is made of copper and zinc (5:1) and similarly, bronze (kanchu) is principally an alloy of copper and tin (4:1). Bell metal (kanchu) ore is a sulphide of tin, copper, and iron. However, bronze and brass may also include small proportions impurities like arsenic, phosphorus, aluminum, manganese, and even silicon. These are beneficial and slow in absorption into the body.

Some more metals like silver and gold articles along with metals like lead, mercury, cadmium and even tin. But they can have some harmful effects in high doses, but their slow absorption at ppm levels – can extend beneficial results too. They also suffer from a drawback, with chronic accumulation- if used for a long time. Here, high lead metal levels-reduce oxygen availability to the body, mercury – a deadly poisonous metal-erodes arteries and similarly cadmium erodes immune system. So, such metals only get added as impurities with beneficial results.

"Hence a cautious approach is needed regarding the use of such toxic inorganic metal salts and some such studies are already in progress even in western nations"

Hence, gold shilajit are considered to be curator of evil effects and bad omens, sliver shilajit- natural is considered to be a brain sharpener and copper shilajit serve as bacilli growth inhibitor. Here bone decorated articles like lamb or cow/buffalo horns, tiger nails, elephant tusks; yak bones- are available near places of worship or nearby markets. Thus, animal bone made as garlands cure bad omens. In routine wear of ornaments, gold or silver or some base metals in hand & foot is a common observation in India.

There is another important article on adsorption- desorption of heavy metal ions by S.P. Misra (current sci, <u>102</u>, p601, 2014, review article) wherein teak tree bark powder, rice husk, etc., were investigated. The results are interesting suggesting chromium can desorb lead & zinc ions and in turn chromium can be desorbed by normal alkali-s.

Here chromium-based treatments are prevalent in China to reduce cancer risks due to high atomic radiations. Ayurvedics use the tree bark or its ash, with excellent results.

5.iv. Daily Needs

What are the daily requirements of the body for an average human being?

Calcium: The most vital ion of daily requirement is calcium. It is divalent and the ore size is less than potassium and thus has free permeability into each cell with metals like manganese, magnesium and sodium. Potassium is a captive ion in a human cell and its loss means destruction a cell.

It is calcium meddling as calmodulin release insulin and it is calcium that gives strength to bones and teeth. Increased calcium levels even reduce blood pressure. Calcium also helps vit. D absorption by the body. Here calcium precipitation is also needed by hard tissues like teeth and bones. Calcium is supplemented by milk, pulses, green leafy vegetables, citrus fruits and even milk products. In Betel leaf with calcium basically added to stimulate insulin release from the pancreas.

Indian-pan (plus katha, sugar, elachi, gulkand, grated coconut, and processed supari), serve as a digestive tool and also an insulin releaser. Here katha probably acts like calmodulin by carrying calcium to the site of action and without application of katha excess calcium can create mouth sores also.

Phosphorus: It is phosphates that carry calcium ion into the cell. Absence of phosphates leads to the absence of ATP formation. The cyclic AMP formation means termination of metabolism and even slowing of healing process. But the body is not capable of absorbing inorganic phosphates direct. Hence phosphate salts are given to plants and man consumes such products to get phosphates into his body. Thus, all phosphates must come from natural resources through egg or milk, nuts, fruits, pulses, beans as body needs @ one gram/day.

Magnesium: It has scope in every cell and helps in vitamin C absorption. It is again copper – magnesium balance that controls nervous system. In France low magnesium in soil led to high incidence of cancer. In urology it is magnesium ion that has the capacity to break kidney and gall bladder stones. The body needs about 200-400 mg daily. Magnesium is also present in pulses, nuts, leafy vegetables and milk, which are daily needs.

Sodium and potassium: They are present in common salt added for taste. In case of high blood pressure patients, Sindhava salt is recommended as it is richer in potassium in comparison to common salt. The blood pressure is determined by the simple ratio of sodium and captive potassium ions in the cells. If a person is metal ion-deficient, he tries to eat even mud (– la Krishna in his childhood). Potassium is vital for soft tissues and is present in banana, leafy vegetables, nuts, pulses, paprika and the body needs @ 0.5- 1 gm of both sodium and potassium ions.

Zinc: It controls more than 300 enzymatic reactions being rapidly reactive. Though one needs only 20-30 mg per day, its absence means loss of taste, and its absence also means delay in healing. Even a human reproductive activity cannot be accomplished if zinc is absent in testis. It is said that ayurvedics give tin salts here to stimulate these actions. These zinc salts also help hair growth and its deficiency can lead to baldness or hair fall. It is deficiency that leads to higher iron and copper utilization in the body, thereby reducing less oxygen absorption in lungs and also can lead to undesirable cholesterol levels. Pumpkin seeds are rich in zinc and zinc cures even mental sickness. It is also available in spinach, peas, nuts, seeds, pulses, & brown rice.

Iron: The body needs it in petty amounts like 16-20 mg daily. When the blood breaks up the iron ion becomes free and mostly it is reabsorbed by the body. Iron as Fe^{2+} and Fe^{3+} contribute to the respiratory process. It as trivalent gets circulated into the body and returns to lungs as divalent – means oxygen supply to the entire biological actions-anaerobic oxidations in the body. In South India green vegetables find their way in food chain as they are rich in iron and potassium.

Copper: It works as a partner with iron. It is copper that provide vital electric pulse to iron and in turn gets purged out. It is copper deficiency leads to CNS collapse or even anemia. It is copper that increases cholesterol levels and also decrease HDL levels. It even reduces bacterial infestation into the body and ayurveda recommend it for controlling diseases of nerves like syphilis and venereal diseases. So, copper has tendency to increase blood pressure. It is present in dried legumes, nuts, wheat germs, banana and even honey.

Iodine: In fact, it is WHO recommendation of iodized salt to reduce the incidence of thyroid problems. There are minor ions like selenium and chromium. It is chromium that is lost in injury during operation. It also helps in sugar conversion of fatty acids to cholesterol. It is manganese that helps utilization of vitamin B & E and its over dose reduce brain activity even. The last, yet important ion is selenium that sweeps all nodes inside the body and keeps liver active. All these metals come through whole grains, nuts etc., and there is no need to add extra.

Here, even siddha or Aamchi system or even Unani system of medicine use maximum metallic ions in the treatment. But for using them, even homeopathy or siddha or Unani restrict some sour foods by experience. I find the use of compounded mercury in treatments like (rasa-rath of Divya pharmacy-which I was prescribed in mg levels), Rasa sindhur or kajjali etc.,- are used even today.

5. v. Crude Metal Preparations-(Ayurveda) Some are Listed below

A. Abhrakam (mica, @50% Si and other major metals Al and Mg, Fe);

B. talakam (haritala, yellow arsenic);

C. hingulam (ingilicam, cinnabar, red substance – mercury rich);

D. manisila (realgar arsenic sulphide);

E. navasaram (white solid, ammonium chloride);

F. sindhava salt or potassium rich sodium chloride;

G. veligaram (tankana, borax); h. gandhakam or Sulphur;

H. yavakshar (alkali prepn. Out of barli or rice);

I. Yasuda (zinc);-are some important materials in Indian medicine. Thus, the question arises such as how to prepare Bhasma out of them. Some crude procedures are as below.

- Naga bhasma: take lead flakes in a mud basin, heat it slowly till it melts and go on adding black pepper beads till all liquid totally lead dissolves. Here excess pepper a couple of beads does not matter as it burns in no time in a hot vessel to give a fine ash.

- Rasa bhasma: Taken clean distilled mercury, which used to be done in earthen ware in old days. Now take cleaned mercury in a pingani vessel (ceramic lined vessel), and added concentrated sulphuric acid dropwise till all mercury is dissolved and reduced to a powder. Leave overnight and now dilute the acid and collect the rasa bhasma. Sometimes it needs three or five purifications before finally accepted as a drug.

- Tamra bhasma: The copper coin is put in go- panca-kam (five cow products- called go-pancakam- milk, curd, ghee, urine, & cow dung) for one hour and repeated with fresh mixture go-pancakam twice, to get clean copper coin.

- Copper coin can also be purified by soaking in svarasa of drumstick tree and burning it. Now takeout the coin and repeat this process seven times to get cleaned copper coin.

- Copper Bhasma: This copper coin is soaked in vakudu root crushed fluid and applied gajaputam to get white bhasma.

- Purification of tamra bhasma: the tamra-bhasma is mixed with castor oil and such a paste is put in a wheat powdered cup (cup made of wet atta) and this mixture is sealed with atta paste from all sides, with no air in it. Now, it is subjected to gajaputam.

- Rasa vanga (tin) bhasma: if one is losing grip on indriyas, give rasa vanga – bhasma. It is prepared with kali mirch 1 tola, sunthi 0.4 tola, dalchini 0.4 tola, loang 28 no., jeera 0.4 tola, revand chini 0.4 tola, tanikai 1 tola, karakkai 1 tola, japatri 1 tola, jaji kai 0.4 tola, Chhota-elachi 1 tola, tava ksheeram 3 tola, seep one tola, tagaram 3 tola, mercury 1 tola,

Procedure: Take tagaram in a mud donga and heat till it melts. Now put mercury and heat with shaking so that tin dissolves to give fine particles. Take all herbs as burnt ash and pass-through muslin. Now add entire herb burnt ash to the tin-mercury combination and also some herb powder as such. All will get burnt and continue the heating with shaking. Later all contents are cooled and finely grinded for several hours. Finally, by using tava ksheeram (sterile & heated milk) and muslin filtered ash are mixed to make a goli and dried in shade. It is given as directed by a physician. Note that it in high doses or not well compounded material can be fatal or cause several side effects. Hence, these are repeatedly purified as putam in Sanskrit and are given with ghee or butter milk.

It is noteworthy to note that zinc or lead or tin or mercury are used in extreme cases like cancer (arbuda), or severe worm infections.

In my observation, lead salts benefit joint pains and also some diabetic patients, tin salts benefit aphrodisiac combinations, copper salts help in the skin affections, zinc salts help digestive tract in the body and finally mercury salts like Rasa-sindhur halt every type of infections. The old ayurvedic practitioners used these poisons as curable complexes, including arsenic preparations. Yet all metal ions have their share of negative affects too.

"Though, I have hinted about crude metallic preparations, I have little knowledge in this subject. Their purification and improves of potency with a number of putam (purifications)- is a huge well-defined subject.

This is done by hand-made cow dung cakes (called pidaka) in fire (putam)- is an exclusive ayurvedic specialty! Here, not all salt preparations are covered- but small hint given. But, if bacilli expand beyond control in an exponential way, to curb them., an increased lead, copper, arsenic or mercury complexes (– some of these were even patented by ICMR in early '50's).

Thus, if there is a sudden bacterial/chemical attack- may bring back patented mineral complexes and also no rescue except use of age- old mercury or arsenic based preparations. To date Unami and homeopathy practice the use of arsenic and other metal combinations.

Thus, metal salts of arsenic, copper & selenium are known bactericides and fungicides, where magnesium, manganese, and calcium act as moderators cum diluents.

Experiments are going using mercury in Canada. and more nations. To resist radiation, chromium salts are administered in China. If choice is between life or death, there is no alternative then and so can be used.

The modern physician prescribes tablets, like Glacex, Cobadex, Zevit, zincovit, revital, etc., medicines-rich in minerals and vitamins.

How the next level of disease treatments can be handled using herbs?

Do herbs have the potency to tackle or cure or reduce impact of diseases. Let us look into in part-II Health.

Health - Herbs & Spices as Medicines

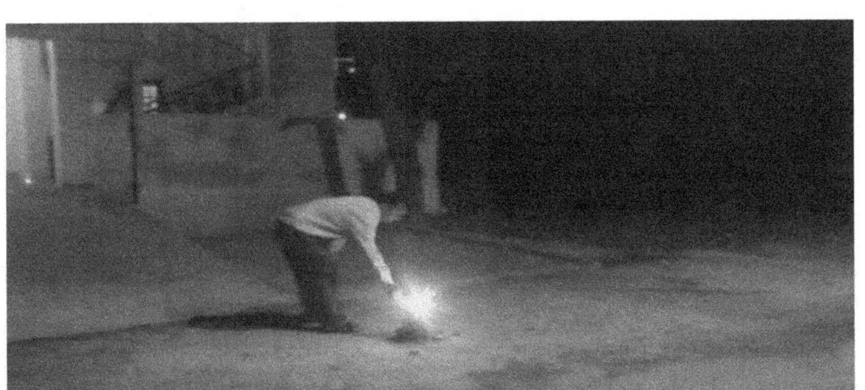

Front of the house- with land barren above (2009- Diwali); Photo below is of 2023, with mango & ganneru etc. plants.

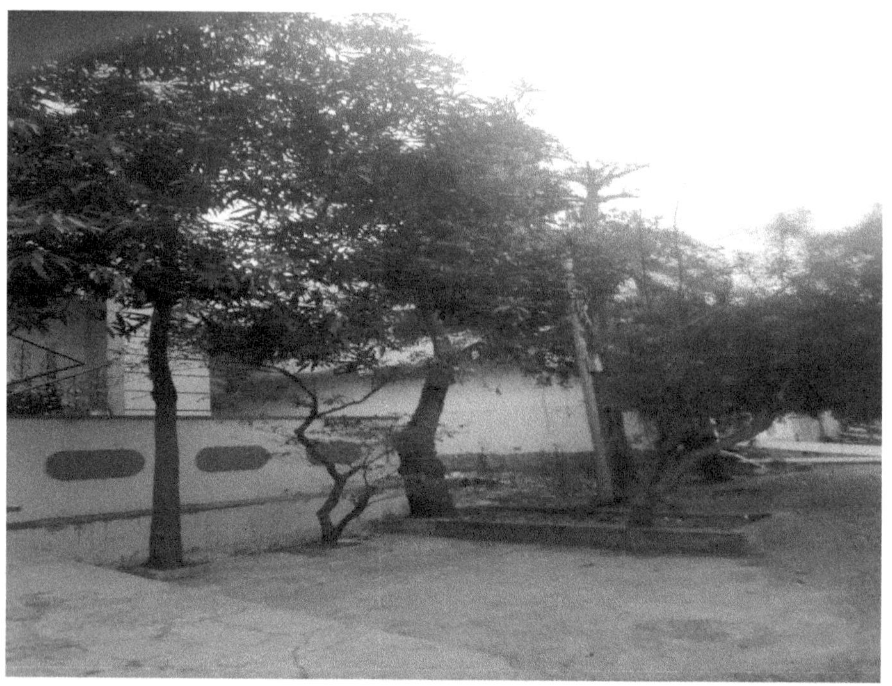

6. Treatment or Chikitsa (with Ayurvedic Herbs)

Whenever a disease is struck, it is said that the body has a defense mechanism to fight every type of disease and only supplements are needed to fight.

Man needs food for regular nourishment and survival, which is depicted in ayurveda as dosha. Man needs a solution for the digestive problems as food is a necessity. In home therapy, we have witnessed the use of vegetables, cereals to treat hunger and recover from simple problems.

There can be more severe problems that need a solution. How are these problems arriving into the body?

The theory suggests that thsy can be seen as

A. Sancaya: in a state of accumulation;

B. Prokop: Stage of eruption-like rapid rash formation etc.,

C. Prasara: it is ia a state of spreading;

D. Stana samsraya: localized to a place;

E. Vyatka: manifestation or expression of a disease is visible;

F. Bheda: changes (chronic/permanent) damage due to pathological changes.

G. Injury treatment needs sadhana (cleaning & nursing).

I appreciate every correction at every level, if I am wrong.

Many procedures in the later stages implemented to cure are cumber sum, but needed.

6.d.i. These are listed below-starting from five procedures (panca-karma). They are Langhana (fast),- Vamana (omitting), – virechana (loose motions through purgation), or enema therapy or with daily exercises, long walk etc.,-Siro-virechana-(nasya or smoking spices or sweating head etc.,). Thus, Langhana causes- depletion of body resources; Svedana- hot bath and tie a thick blanket to generate sweat; Brimhana- Nourishing; to supplement dhatus – like milk juices; Snehana-Application of salt, pepper, pulses, butter etc., on skin; The treatment is through Pachana (using digestive stimulants); deepana (hot blanket); kshut (hunger control); Thrit (increased intake of water & laxatives); yama (exercises); Athapa (exposure to sunlight or infrared); Maruta- elimination of digestive gases, etc.

Even the human epidermis consists of six layers in ayurveda like Apsara, Purnima etc., (ayurvedic conference in 1984, GAU, Jamnagar). They have defined the skin thickness to be directly proportional to the grain (vriha) – regularly consumed by us-with a formula. How many years such studies on vriha had been done-long back?

d.ii. Safe Herbal Combinations

The ayurvedic scholars grouped like-minded herbs for use in treatments. Here ayurvedic physicians classified them into fifty groups of compatible medicinal herbs (gana-s)- based upon their use. They also suggested some simple & safe combinations in ayurveda:

1. Trikatu:- (vata, kapha, pitta haratvam). Trikatu is a combination of black pepper, long pepper, dried ginger.

2. Trifala: (the three rejuvenators),- amla, haritaki and vibhitaki.

3. Trijataka: (three digestives), Chhota elachi, tvak (dalchini), tej Patra (Biryani masala).

4. Trimada: (three powerful killers): citraka (leadwort), musta (Cyperus rotundas), vidanga (Embelia ribes).

If one looks into Charak Samhita, there are many more combinations like chaturjataka, panca-bhadra and also many multi herbal combinations- that can handle basic diseases. For example, black pepper is present in more than 100 combinations & used for a variety of diseases as it augments treating power of the combination.

d.iii. Ayurvedic Extraction Methods

Some old procedures in ayurveda are presented below. The same procedure can have multiple names & are closer to modern methods.

1. Maceration: A coarsely powdered drug is placed in a Stoppered container with solvent and allowed to stand at room temperature for three days with occasional shaking. Then mixture is strained and extract collected.

2. Percolation: This is used for the preparation of tinctures and fluid extracts in cold or at room temperature with 95% alcohol.

3. Infusions: Infusion is suggested to be made of maceration with cold or boiling water for a short time and filtered, the filtrate is called infusion, and can be consumed as such through slow sip or with honey.

4. Hima: If infusion is in cold conditions, it is called hima. Here the cold infusion in which, dried and coarsely powdered plant material, is soaked with water for some time and squeezed with muslin. Only sugars and inorganics mostly slip fast into water.

5. Digestion: during cold maceration, if mild to moderate heating is done, it is digestion.

6. Phanta: If plant is crushed and hot infusion is obtained with boiling water & concentrated. (Like jaggery; Panta in Telugu means crop or final product).

7. Decoction or kawath: Generally, it is made up of one pint (@473ml) of water with 30grams (one Oz.) of finely chopped material. It is boiled (in some cases, a time frame is given- lest some herbs can tend to be toxic), cooled and filtered. The decoction can be kept for 72 hours in refrigerated conditions. If the water volume is reduced to 1:4 from 1:16 levels and squeezed- called quath or kawath.

8. Syrup: If the decoction of the drug is concentrated further to 10% the original volume, with heating. To a pint of such an extract add 2-4 table-spoon-full (TSF) glycerin and 2-4 TSF honey later for stability. Here 16 TSF fluids makes one pint.

9. Tinctures: In case syrup is to be made from tinctures instead the plant material, the tincture prepared from herb: alcohol- (1:5 or 1:10). In certain cases, it is vigorously stirred in a blender and kept in closed container & later shaken – at least twice a day for fourteen days. The mixture is prepared with 40 % of sterile water and

    60% glycerin. This mixture (15) parts is diluted with honey ten parts and carefully stir the liquid and preserved. Sometimes extracts as tinctures is added to whisky/brandy and given to patients.

10. The concentrated plant extracts are treated with 65% sugar solution and stored as syrup or murabba (plant material as

cooked lumps in sugar syrup or can be converted to candy or jam.

11. Swarasa: (Plant juices) expeller extraction like sugar cane, orange, apple, pineapple, carrot etc., or alternatively, the fresh plant material is crushed and juice collected by expeller or through muslin, to get juice, concentrated to viscous forms and made up with glycerin (1:5 v/v) for storage.

12. Hot extraction and powders: Continuous Soxhlet extraction is a modern technique. A fresh plant material can decompose, but, the alcoholic extracts can be stored- as thick fluid or even to a dry powder form with additives.

13. 13.Satwa: Hot aqueous/fluid extracts are dried in shade to give a dry powder called satwa(e.g guduchi stawa). Milk is spray dried- a modern technique.

14. Fermentation: It is always done in an earthen vessel. Some medicinal preparations like Asava and Arista, adopt fermentation.

15. Oils: The plant material is directly heated in oil (1:100 or 1:10) to get an essential oil-based extract for external application.

    Ear drops: In case you need a sloppy fluid, take the powdered and dried herb, add olive oil in a ratio 1:5 and keep warm to 100^0 F (or 60^0c) for ten days, which is filtered and stored as ear drops or nasal drops. I use garlic loves- boiled sesame oil, cooled & filtered for ear-ache. Such oils have no expiry date on their use.

16. Ointment: Even the above oil can be made ointment using beeswax; powdered plant material is directly added into olive oil, stir well in a pestle mortar for half an hour or mildly warm,

later bee wax (2: 1) added to it by heating to 500. It is stored in a bottle with lid to serve as an ointment, for external application.

17. Kalka or Poultice:-wet bolus- wherein crushed plant material is used as a paste or as such.

18. Anjana: Take ghee in a container and into it kept a wick dried of desired plant extract and burnt the wick. Keep a plate above and collect the anjana settled on the plate above. Applied to eyes also.

19. The solids can be: Anjana, churna, mansapotli, kshara, gutika, guda, dhumravati, puplika, prithuka, mandura, modaka, Rasa-kriya, vati, varti, shashkuli, saktu, Bhasma, Ras-aushadhi all are different names given to the solid products which differ in processing and use. See more in ayurvedic texts.

20. the liquids in ayurveda are with different names like, Taila, ghrita, asava/arishta, arka, hima, swarasa, peya, phanta, Manda, vilepi, Madya — all is ayurvedic terms for different extracts, liquors-names given for different purposes.

21. Fumigation: dhumra Pana (smoking), dhupana (keeping scented smoke), are different procedures of fumigation.

22. Nasya: A nasal suction of fine dust (nasya) into lungs is also a smart technique of activation. The modern physicians also give drugs as capsules, which get broken and sucked through mouth into lungs-in a similar way.

Thus, several Ayurvedic procedures are still valid. With regard to the dosage aspects, an excellent summation is presented in the book – titled "Hand book of domestic medicine and common ayurvedic remedies"- edited by Sh. P.V.N. Kurup (ICMR, 1978).

For example, the dose of swarasa of a herb to one month old child or less is suggested as 1to 3 drops, and that for a child of 1 to 5 years age group as 2 to

23. ml. A six-gram drug when converted to vati, it can become into few mg vati.

d.iv. Spices: One must also

understand that pepper, garlic, sunthi, jeera or ajowan etc., are spices & medicines- entering into blood as a part of food chain. What are they?

The spices are known safe bactericides and fungicides and test results on gram positive and gram-negative bacilli confirm these results. (See references) Spices are also used for flavor & as taste makers in food. But, excess of anything is bad. Though, the number of spices in the world may exceed to 110 to 150 spices, Indians use only a few- that suit a tropical climate. Thus, Indians are also one of the largest producers and consumers of many spices. Even today, about 18 spices are in commercial production and the rest are on import list.

1. Ajowan, Trachyspermum Ammi, Bishop's weed, Ajwain, Yami- Niki, Vamu, Ajowan: Trachyspermum Ammi – seeds; Its aqueous extract is used in children's gripe water and there exists an ayurvedic procedure to produce that water. The fruit possesses stimulant, antispasmodic and carminative properties and is used traditionally as an important remedial agent digestive, antispasmodic, galactagogue, stimulant, carminative, expectorant, atonic dyspepsia, diarrhea, abdominal pains, piles, and bronchial problems. Hence, its seeds are antiseptic,

stomachic, carminative, & used in diarrhea & colic. It has 0. 4% essential oil and its oil contain 60% thymol.

2. Ajmodaka, Trachyspermum roxbughianum, Ajmod or Wild celery seeds/Radhuni; Its aromatic dried fruits, like its close relative ajwain, are often used in Bengali cuisine but are rarely used in the rest of India. The fresh leaves are used as a herb in Thailand and it is used medicinally in Myanmar. The small dried fruit seeds are similar in appearance to those of ajwain, celery, and caraway.

    Because of their similarity in both appearance and flavor, it is often confused or substituted with celery seed. It is a very strong spice, with a characteristic smell similar to parsley and taste similar to celery. A couple of pinches can easily overpower a curry and widely used in Bengali cuisine.

3. Aniseed: Pimpinella anisum, fruits: Velayati saunf, Chhotii saunf, Star anise, Fennel, Aniseed, Saunf – It is mild expectorant,stimulating, carminative, diuretic, diaphoretic, in asthma powders, in veterinary medicine.; It is one of the oldest medicinal plants. It is an annual grassy herb with 30–50 cm high, white flowers, and small green to yellow seeds. The aniseeds are antimicrobial, antifungal, antiviral, antioxidant, muscle relaxant and analgesic. The fruits are also anticonvulsant, diuretic, carminative, prevents flatulence & colic. The seeds contain 0.5%, essential oil with anethole- being 90%. The essential oils also contain chavicol and alpha-phenyl acetone.

4. Tamarind, Tamarindus indica (fruit): Cinta, Sirimanu, – Refrigerant,digestive, carminative,laxative, antiscorbutic,febrifuge, ophthalmic useful in gastropathy, datura poisoning, alcoholic intoxication, scabies, constipation;

Tintrini, tamarind, amli, imli, ambli or Tamarind- is derived from the Arabic- 'Tamir-e-Hind'. Ripe tamarind pods or mature pods are brown or brownish-black colored fruits which contain hard red-black seeds. Its leaves fresh are consumed as such or even cooked with lentil and consumed.

The fruit is laxative and is an excellent remedy for sluggish bowel movement and it lower the levels of bad cholesterol (LDL) thereby promoting healthy cardiovascular health, this because of the presence of phenols, antioxidants beneficial for levels of HDL. Flowering leaves of tamarind are crushed to extract juice. This juice is a home remedy for piles. Tamarind contains tartaric and other acid derivatives along with minerals. Tamarinds seeds are mixed with turmeric paste are used as a treatment for inflammation and is used as a traditional medicine for jaundice. Root and bark infusions of tamarind are used as an alternative treatment for leprosy.

5. Black pepper, Piper nigrum (fruit): Golmirich, Kali mirch, Vellaja, Marica, Miriyalu, Milagu, Peppercorn; used in spicy foods as curative and also in medicine as marica. It is Anthelmintic, carminative, antiperiodic, diuretic, digestive, emmenagogue, rubefacient, stimulant, stomachic, used in fever, asthma, cough, dyspepsia, flatulence, arthritis. Dried fruits of Piper nigrum (black pepper) are commonly used in gastrointestinal disorders. Its purified form piperine (or spice as such) is a proven bioavailability stimulator for many drugs – as depicted in the award. The aim of this study was to rationalize the medical use of pepper and its principal alkaloid, piperine, in constipation and diarrhea using in vitro and in vivo assays. Black pepper corns are rich in minerals,- like potassium, calcium, zinc, manganese, iron, and magnesium. Pepper

corns are a good source of many anti- oxidant vitamins such as vitamin-C and vitamin-A. The fruit is aromatic, stimulant, dyspepsia, arthritis, used in cholera, fevers & vertigo; anti-pyretic in malaria as alternative, cure arthritis, sore throat, piles, skin diseases, clavacin, piperine, piperettine present in them more than 5 to 11% in these species.

6. White pepper, Piper cubeba: Chavika, Sevasu, Cubeb, Kababchini, White pepper, Cubed, tailed pepper, Java pepper; Tailed Pepper is perennial flowering vine in the family Piperaceae. The fruits are gathered before they are ripe, and carefully dried. They are aromatic,cure hemorrhoids, stimulant, carminative and useful in cough and cold. The cubeb was frequently used in the form of cigarettes for asthma. The dried cubeb berries contain piperine, alpha thujone, germacrene, & alpha and beta cubebins.

7. Maga, Piper longum: Long Pepper, Tippili, Ushna, Chapla, Kana, Pimpli, Pippali, or Pippallu; it is expectorant, diuretic, tonic, purgative, stomachic, digestive, antiseptic, used in bronchitis, fever, asthma indigenous to North-eastern and Southern India and Sri Lanka, the dried or unripe fruit is alterative, tonic, fruit/root antidote to snakebite. The decoction of immature fruits is used in chronic bronchitis, cough, & cold. The immature fruits are soft and they relieve cough on chewing.

8. Malabar Tamarind, Garcinia cambogia: Garcinia Fruit, Brindle berry, Gamboge, Velayati imli, Erda, Kudampuli, Gummi-gutta, Pot tamarind; When Garcinia is taken 30-60 minutes before the meal, the excess carbohydrates are converted to abdominal fats. HCA {(-) hydroxy-citric acid}-decreases the supply of acetyl-CoA- through inhibition of ATP-citrate-lyase

activity. It also accelerated the glucose catabolism and energy metabolism, which eventually reduced fat accumulation. It thus inhibits the formation of fatty acids and hence less fat is available to the cells for storage. HCA also reduces appetite. Over-the-counter, the weight loss supplements usually offer HCA in dosages of 250 to 1,000 mg 3 times daily. It also cures inflammation of the stomach, gastric ulcers, reduces acidity. Its fruit is rich in hydro-citric acid is consumed as condiment in many countries. It is called Malabar tamarind or kudam puli in Kerala & used as a substitute to tamarind in sambar masala. Garcinia fruit is also infused in tea although it is bitter and a small amount of it in conjunction with other herbs to make it palatable. Garcinia extract may be consumed as a capsule. Another is Mangosteen (Garcinia mangostana) is available as a fresh fruit and its fruit pulp is sweet & juicy with a very pleasant aroma and useful in sugar reduction.

9. Kokum, Garcinia indica: Raktapooraka, Vrikshamla, Wild mangosteen, Murgal, Punumpuli; Garcinia indica, a plant in the mangosteen family (Clusiaceae), commonly known as kokum, is a fruit-bearing tree that has culinary, pharmaceutical, and industrial uses.

Garcinia indica is an anti-oxidant rich fruit used in the name of Vrikshamla in Ayurveda. Its fruits are green when unripe. Only ripe dark red colored fruit is useful for medicinal purposes.

Fruit antiscorbutic, cooling, cholagogue, emollient, demulcent; bark- astringent; its oil used to cure skin affections. Kokum butter juice prepared from its fruits is a famous coolant summer juice and widely used for loosing body weight also.

10. Amlavetasa, Garcinia pedunculata: Sohdanei, Bar thekera; the bark is thick and corky. The plant is cultivated for local use as a medicine and food. Its fruit is roundish with a diameter @ 10 cm, with juicy interior & edible. It is an evergreen tree-Garcinia mangostana or the more familiar purple mangosteen.

    The fruit prevents scurvy (antiscorbutic). The ripe fruit is either eaten cooked or raw or the ripe or raw fruits sliced, sun-dried and preserved. In the state of Assam such slices are used for preparing delicacies. Sohdanei is also known to be rich in antioxidants.

11. Naga Valli, Piper betle: Betel leaf plant, Saptashira, Pan, Vitika, Tambul, Nagvallaril; the betel (Piper betle) is the leaf of a vine belonging to the Piperaceae family, which includes pepper and kava. It is valued both as a mild stimulant and for its medicinal properties.

    The betel plant is an evergreen perennial, with glossy heart-shaped leaves and white catkin. The leaf is carminative, stimulant, digestive, juice of leaves, put even into eyes to relieve cerebral congestions & night blindness. The leaf is employed with honey as a remedy for cough and root is used for anti-implantation effect.

12. Caper, Capparis spinosa: Himsra, Cabra, Mullukattari, Caper bush, Flinders rose, a perennial plant. It is best known for the edible flower buds (capers), and the fruit (caper berries), both are consumed or pickled. It also reduces the impact of high radiation levels. The fruits are diuretic, aspirant, expectorant, emmenagogue, & tonic. It is also used in rheumatism, gout, afflictions of liver and spleen. Suppliers: Afghanistan or Indian subcontinent.

13. Caraway, Carum carvi: Alcaravea, Meridian fennel, Persian cumin, Kala-jeera: It is stomachic,carminative, anthelmintic,lactagogue, adjuvant/corrective for nauseating & griping effects of medicines. It is a biennial plant and is native to Asia, Europe and Africa. Suppliers: India, Europe, Persia; Caraway is valued for dyspepsia, colic and flatulence. Caraway is also used as intestinal diuretic, antiseptic and anti-inflammatory. It is traditionally used to stimulate appetite, & digestion and also known to boost the immune system. It is used for a variety of gastro-intestinal disorders including heartburn, stomach spasm and digestion.

14. Cardamom, Elettaria cardamomum (small), Elam: Ancha, Elachi, Ela chi, Elaki, Ala, Bahula, Bhadra Ila, Bhringa-parnika, Chhota elachi or Elettaria cardamomum (fruit) – It is an evergreen, perennial ginger-like plant, stimulant, tonic, diuretic, carminative, digestive, expectorant, & cardiotonic. Cardamom is used internally for indigestion, nausea, vomiting and pulmonary disease with copious phlegm. It can be used with a laxative to prevent stomach pain, griping, as well as flatulence. Cardamom is also brought in used to kidney stones and gall stones. Cardamom is used as a flavoring agent in food preparations. It contains formic and acetic acid derivatives, improves sex life, contains manganese, fights anaemia, regulate heart beat & stomachic.

15. Cassia, Cinnamomum cassia, Dalchini: (stem bark) It is astringent, stimulant, carminative, germicidal, tonic, diuretic, carminative, emmenagogue, anti- inflammatory Cinnamon astringent, diuretic, carminative, aphrodisiac, deodorant, expectorant, febrifuge, stomachic.

16. Chinese cinnamon, Cinnamomum aromaticum: Cassia cinnamon, dalchini; cortex; some people *use* it for erectile dysfunction (ED), hernia, bed-wetting and joint pain. Used for confectionary, desserts, pastries, curry and meat. It is aromatic, astringent and carminative, effective in combating digestive disorders, diarrhea and gastroenteritis, as well as stimulating the body. It is anti-oxidant too.

17. True cinnamon, Cinnamomum Zeylanicum: Laurus Cinnamomum, Ceylon Cinnamon; it is the bark was used in food to prevent spoiling. It is used as a spice and aromatic. Traditionally, the bark or oil has been used to combat micro-organisms, diarrhea and Gi tract disorders.

 It is a part of trijataka- a condiment used to digest delicious foods as dalchini is aromatic, astringent and carminative too.

18. Cinnamomum verum, Cinnamon, (stem bark) dalchini; condiment and flavoring material;

19. Dalchini, Cinnamomum sulphuratum: used its bark and leaves like that of the related species, C. zeylanicum, to cure coughs, headaches, spider poison and as a mouth refresher. The bark is useful as medicine and also for preparing agarbathi.

20. Karpuramchettu, Cinnamomum camphora: Camphorwood, Gandhadravya, camphor laurel; Twigs are usually green, but may be tinged with red when young.

 The berries first turn reddish, then ripen to black. Camphor tree can be readily identified by the distinctive odor of a crushed leaf.

Camphor Tree is native to China, Japan, Korea, Taiwan, and adjacent parts of East Asia. It is now cultivated in many parts of the world.

21. Celery, Apium graveolens, Ajmod, Ajwain ka patta, Wild celery, Ajmud; Used for weight loss and even reduce hypertension. It is an aromatic bitter herb which reduces

blood pressure, relieves indigestion, and stimulates the uterus, acts as anti-inflammatory, diuretic and aphrodisiac. Its seeds contain 2-3% essential oils and the oil is antiseptic, tonic, asthma, liver and spleen disorders and emmenagogue. A vegetable with anti-inflammatory, anti-hypertensive actions; Contains citric, iso-citric, fumaric, malic and tartaric acids; Limonene, phthalides, β-selinene, selinene, apiol, type essential oil constituents.

22. Mirchi, Capsicum annum or Capsicum frutescens: Chili pepper, Mirapa, (fruits) – It is digestive,thermogenic, carminative,stimulant, cardiotonic, antipyretic, sudorific, rubefacient & sialagogue; has been used to treat diabetes mellitus in Jamaica. It is a stimulant, cures yellow fever and dyspepsia. Its dried powder is antiseptic, cures even snake bite. The ancient use is for treatment of cough, and sore throat. A weak fruit infusion can be employed as a gargle to treat throat complaints.

The fresh juice applied to the cavity to cure toothache. Poultice of chili powder is used for treating injuries and even rheumatic pains. But more use of chili leads to duodenal ulcers also.

23. Clove, Syzygium aromaticum, Luong, Clove, Karampu, (buds): Refrigerant, ophthalmic, digestive, carminative, stomachic, stimulant, antispasmodic, antibacterial, expectorant,

rubefacient, Aphrodisiac, appetizer, emollient; the dried flower bud is known as laong. It acts as a stimulant and is very useful in relieving problems of spasmodic disorders. It relieves flatulence and stimulates the sluggishness of blood circulation promoting digestion. It is a stimulant, aromatic and used in dyspepsia. Essential oil from clove mainly contained about 87.00% eugenol. Its oil is dental antiseptic.

24. Indian Blackberry, Syzygium cumini (Eugenia jambolana): Jambul, Black Plum, Java Plum, Neredu; black plum or "jamun" is an important medicinal plant in various traditional systems of medicine. It is effective in the treatment of diabetes mellitus, inflammation, ulcers and diarrhea and preclinical studies have also shown it to possess chemo-preventive, radio-protective and anti-neoplastic properties. The plant is rich in compounds containing anthocyanins, glucoside, ellagic acid, iso-quercetin, kaempferol and myricetin. The seeds are claimed to contain alkaloid, jambosine, and glycoside jambolin or antimellin, which halts the diastatic conversion of starch into sugar. The fruit is astringent, useful in diarrhea, biliousness and seeds used in diabetes. The root bark is astringent & used as decoction to gargle. The fruit juice with goat milk cures diarrhea in children. The seed, leaf, bark, and fruit are used to make medicine.

25. Coriander, Coriandrum sativum: (fruit); Dhania, Phadigom, Ulichya;—It is carminative, diuretic, tonic, stimulant, stomachic, refrigerant, aphrodisiac, analgesic, anti-inflammatory. Coriander also acts as an aphrodisiac, discharging urine, removal of phlegm from the bronchial tube and helps in the elimination of catarrhal substances from the body.

Coriander seeds give a feeling of coolness. The juice of the herb is highly beneficial because of the presence of Vitamin A, B,

B2, C and iron. The leaves or herb or even dried seeds are used as a condiment in food, sauces & curries. The oil of the herb is used in medicines. The dried coriander serves as a tonic and stimulant. They make the stomach strong and are known to increase secretion of juices, relieve flatulence as well as reduce fever.

26. Cumin, Cuminum cyminum, Jeera, Safed Zira, Jeeraka, Sveta-jiraka, Zira, Jeelakara: a digestive, carminative, astringent, anti-inflammatory, constipating,diuretic, revulsive, galactagogue, uterine & nerve stimulant.

Suppliers: India, Iran, Lebanon; The seeds have a distinctive flavor and an important spice used in food, stews and soups. It is an ayurvedic medicine used for several diseases of the digestive, respiratory, circulatory and even reproductive system. It is antacid, astringent, anodyne and even diuretic. It also helps in treating disorders, worm infestation, nausea, vomiting, and irritable bowels.

27. Dill, Anethum graveolens, Salapuspi, Satapuspi, Sowa, Surva, Sompa, Sadapa-vittulu: It is Carminative, stomachic, & antipyretic. Fennel Stimulant, carminative, stomachic, emmenagogue, refrigerant, cardiac stimulant, antiemetic, aphrodisiac, anthelmintic.

It has been used in medicine since ancient times and it is a popular herb widely used as a spice and also yields essential oil @0.5%, it is aromatic and is an annual herb. Dill seeds are carminative, stomachic and diuretic. Dill has been used both as food and medicine for a very long time.

The Roman gladiators used the burned seeds on wounds to speed up healing. Dill is used as an appetizer. It is believed to stimulate peristaltic motion of the intestine. It is used as an herbal remedy for insomnia.

Monoterpenes and flavonoids are present in dill and its essential oils are germicidal or bactericidal in nature. It is a spice with healing properties.

28. 28. Fennel, Foeniculum vulgare, (fruit): Saunf, Common fennel, sweet fennel, Sompu, saunf, Pedda-jilakarra; – It is a part of Indian/-Chinese medicine- digestive, mouth freshener; Fennel is a well-known and important medicinal and aromatic plant widely used as carminative, digestive, lactagogue and diuretic and in treating respiratory and gastro-intestinal disorders.

It is an insect repellant and aether-oleum is vermicide too. It is also lactagogue, diuretic & useful in treating respiratory and gastrointestinal disorders. Fennel has been used as an herbal remedy for poisoning and stomach conditions.

29. Fenugreek, Trigonella foenum – gracecum: Methika, Methre, Methi, Vendayam: Carminative,tonic, aphrodisiac, emollient, antibacterial, used in vomiting, fever, anorexia, colonitis; Its seeds are tonic, carminative, aphrodisiac and anti-diabetic. Even its leaf is coolant. Its seeds are known to contain metformin & trigonelline,- the drug given to reduce blood sugar levels. Fenugreek has been used in food items as a flavoring agent since ancient times. The leaves and the seeds are known for their medicinal value. It is pungent & aromatic.

Uses of Fenugreek like Allergies, loss of appetite, catarrh/bronchial, reduce cholesterol, anti-diabetic, gas and gastric disorders, lung infections, mucus excessive, throat/sore, abscesses, anemia, asthma, boils, body odor and bronchitis.

Seed of fenugreek also contain flavonoids like quercetin, rutin, vitexin etc.,

30. Curry leaf, Murraya koneigii, Karivepa: (leaf); The leaf is dried and powdered as it is astringent, anthelmintic, febrifuge, stomachic, appetizing, carminative, constipating, anti-inflammatory, antiseptic; it is useful in skin affections, ulcers and even in diarrhea. Suppliers, India, Burma, Sri Lanka;

31. Garlic, Allium sativum, (bulb/its clove); Lasson, Allium, Stinking rose, Porrum sativum, Vellulli; Anti-hyperlipidemic, anti-fungal, tonic, rubefacient, stimulant, thermogenic, and aphrodisiac, used in cough, asthma, and cardiopathy;- Suppliers: Argentina, India, China and many others; Used in the treatment of high cholesterol and high blood pressure.

Traditionally, it has been used for its antiseptic and antibacterial properties, as well as for treating the common cold, upper respiratory tract infections, mild bronchitis, and rhinitis, and to relieve cough and congestion. Other potential uses include treatment of atherosclerosis, enlarged prostate, diabetes, gastrointestinal (GI) disorders. Used as an antiseptic & also acts like an antibiotic. It is useful in skin diseases, colic, carminative, fevers, cough and intermittent fevers.

32. Onion, Allium cepa: Pyaz, Garden onion, Palandu; The onion is also known as the bulb onion or common onion, is a vegetable and is the most widely cultivated species of the genus Allium. It is a stimulant, diuretic, expectorant, aphrodisiac, contains Sulphur compounds like garlic and mustard but in lesser concentration.

33. Welsh onion, Allium fistulosum: Japanese bunching onion, Allium fistulosum is only known in cultivation and probably

originated in north-western China. It was derived from the wild Allium altaicum Pall. It occurs in Siberia and Mongolia, where it is occasionally collected as a vegetable for local use. It is used to improve the functioning of internal organs and the metabolism, for the prevention of cardiovascular disorders, and to prolong life. It is further reported to improve eyesight, and to enhance recovery from common colds, headaches, wounds and festering sores. The weight of 1000 seeds is 2.2–2.5 g, & cultivated.

34. Ginger, Zingiber officinale: (rhizome), Adrakh, Allam, Viswabheshaja, Nagara, Inge; Allam is digestive, carminative, emollient, appetizer, stomachic, rubefacient, anodyne, expectorant, anthelmintic, stimulant; Ginger is well known as a remedy for travel sickness, nausea and indigestion and is used for wind, colic, irritable bowel, loss of appetite, chills, cold, flu, poor circulation, menstrual cramps, dyspepsia (bloating, heartburn,flatulence), indigestion and gastrointestinal problems.

    Suppliers: India, Jamaica, Nigeria, and Sierra Leone; It has pot oxalate 0.5 to 0.8 % & essential oil gingerine, gingerol, all about 1.3 % in it. The rhizome is rich in antioxidant compounds like beta-sitosterol palmitate, isovanillin, glycol Mon palmitate, hexa-cosanoic acid 2,3-dihydroxypropyl ester, maleimide-5-oxime, p- hydroxy- benzaldehyde, adenine, 6-gingerol, and 6-shogaol etc.,

35. Cardamom – large, Amomum subulatum, Black cardamom, Bari ilaichi, large cardamom, Nepal cardamom; (fruit)-Hypnotic, appetizer, astringent to bowels, tonic to heart and liver.

Suppliers: Nepal, India; Black cardamom has a fresh and aromatic aroma. Camphor is easily discernible in its odor. The seeds contain 3% of an essential oil, which is dominated by 1,8-cineol (typically 70%). Smaller and variable amounts of α-terpinyl acetate, limonene, terpinene, terpineol and sabinene have also been reported. Aromatic, digestive, useful in neuralgia, gonorrhea, & aphrodisiac; oil from seeds applied on eyelids to allay inflammation; used in scorpion bite.

36. 36. Mint, Mentha piperita, Velayati pudina, Peppermint leaf: (leaf or terminal shoot) – Stimulant, stomachic, carminative, antiseptic, digestive, antispasmodic, used to prevent vomiting, skin diseases, amenorrhea, dental caries; Peppermint is a hybrid mint, a cross between water mint and spearmint, Peppermint is commonly thought to soothe or treat symptoms such as nausea, vomiting, abdominal pain, indigestion, irritable bowel, and bloating; pudina contains 0.5% essential oil, stimulant, carminative, stomachic, prevent vomiting.

37. Mustard, Brassica campestris or. Brassica nigra: (seed), Avalu (Telugu), Rai (Gujarati), Sorse (Bengali), Mohori (Marathi), Sarson (Hindi); – Thermogenic, anodyne, anti-inflammatory, carminative, digestive, anthelmintic, sudorific, tonic, emetic, used in vomiting, abdominal colic, dyspepsia, flatulence, skin diseases; Seeds used in exacerbations, and tumors.

Brassica oil is used in cooking and during body and hair massages. Seed cake, locally known as Khal or whole plant is given as fodder to increase milk production. These crushed pods are then spread on a piece of cloth and placed in sunlight for 7-8 h. After drying, the crushed pods are removed from the cloth and again ground for 3-4 min.

This powder (pakhi) is then stored in a glass bottle and given to patients suffering from leucorrhea, body weakness, menstrual disorder, greets, and internal pain. The roots and seeds are stomachic. The seeds are used in rheumatism, stiff neck and in dengue fever as external applicant to cure the diseases.

38. Jaiphal, Myristica fragrans, (aril/seed kernel): Mace, Nutmeg, Jatiphala, Jatiphalam, Jatikosha, Jatipatri, Jatipatra; It is astringent, sweet, thermogenic, aphrodisiac, anti-inflammatory, anodyne, deodorant, digestive, expectorant, narcotic, anticonvulsant, antiseptic, constipating – Suppliers: Grenada, Indonesia, India; Mace is often used as a spice in cooking. The herb can help lower blood pressure, sooth a stomach ache and control diarrhea. The oil is a potent brain booster as it increases concentration and relieves stress. Mace is an excellent liver tonic. It dissolves kidney stones and prevents infection.

The herb is also beneficial for the heart as it stimulates blood circulation. Mace's anti-inflammatory properties are used to treat joint and muscle aches. Its seeds are carminative, stomachic, and useful in flatulency, nausea and vomiting. It contains saponins. Its essential oil is rich in alpha pinene, camphene, myrcene and myristicin also besides many more compounds.

39. Bay leaf: Laurus nobilis (leaf) – It is stimulant in sprains, narcotic & used like tejpatta.

Tejpatra, Cinnamomum Tamala, Tamalaja, Talis Patri, Indian bay leaf, Malabar leaf, Indian cassia, or Malabathrum; Carminative, used in colic, diarrhea. Bark is aromatic and used for treating gonorrhea, leaves – flavoring agent and appetizer.

It contains phellandrene, eugenol etc., Its bark contains cinnamaldehyde.

40. Parsley, Petroselinum crisp mum, Prajamoda, Achiu, Ajmod, Curly leaf parsley: (leaf) – Stimulant, diuretic, carminative, emmenagogue, antipyretic, anti-inflammatory, emetic, aphrodisiac, alexipharmic, refrigerant; It is believed that Parsley was used by Romans to relieve problems of the eye and also as a tonic that helped in increasing the strength of the Roman gladiators. The herb contains large quantities of Vitamin A and C. This plant is native to the southern parts of Europe. Its dried ripe fruit used for amenorrhea. It contains some major constituents like juniper camphor,

41. Poppy, Papaver somniferum, (seed); Poppy seed; Khas-khas, Gasagasalu: – Poppy seeds expectorant, sudorific, sedative, nervine tonic, constipating, aphrodisiac; used in internal hemorrhages, diarrhea, dysentery.

42. Rosemary, Rosmarinus officinalis: (leaf/terminal shoot) – Astringent, nervine tonic, stomachic, antibacterial, protistocidal, rubefacient, used in head aches and hardy menstruation; Rosemary is applied for preventing and treating baldness. It is also used for treating circulation problems, gum disease (gingivitis) and toothache. Useful on skin to treat eczema, muscle pain, or pain along the sciatic nerve, and chest wall.

Rosemary is a perennial plant,- used to alleviate muscle pain, improve memory, boost the immune and circulatory system, and promote hair growth.

43. Salvi tulasi, Salvia officinalis: Sauja, Sauge, Swage, Anti-bacterial, (leaf) – Sage is a mild tonic, astringent, carminative,

deodorant, insecticidal, antipyretic, used in gingivitis, gargles, dentifrice, mouthwash; It is rich in vitamins, minerals and anti-oxidants. It is used as salad and also may reduce blood sugar levels.

44. Tropical sage, Salvia spendens: Moroklei, Red Salvia, Scarlet sage; Salvia spendens is widely used in Indian traditional medicine & have been cultivated worldwide for use in folk medicines and for culinary purposes. Sage tea used as a gargle for sore throat and as an aid to digestion. Sage is also used for the value of the natural estrogens and uterotonic.

    It contains polyphenols in its leaves. There are many powerful active constituents- found to be antioxidant. A sage tea can be made by steeping one teaspoon of dried S. officinalis (any variety) in one cup of hot water for about 10 minutes.

45. Star anise of China, Illicium verum- fructus, Star anise, Thakkolam, Anashuppu, Chakra phool; (fruit), Chinese star anise – Astringent, carminative, deodorant, expectorant, digestive; Some people inhale star anise to treat the respiratory tract congestion. It is also stomachic and carminative. It is also used in flavoring foods and beverages. It is also used for easing child birth and also to increase the flow of breast milk. It is widely used in many countries.

46. Saffron, Crocus sativus (flower), Kumkumapuvu – Stimulant, tonic, stomachic, aphrodisiac, anodyne, anti-spasmodic, emmenagogue, diuretic, laxative, used in bronchitis, fever, epilepsy, discoloration of skin; it is used widely in tropical and subtropical countries for a variety of purposes.

    One of our most popular fall-planted bulbs is the Crocus Sativus. Due to the amount of labor involved in harvesting, saffron is one of the world's most expensive spices. The stigmas, and sometimes the petals, are also used in medicine. Saffron is used for asthma, cough, sore throat, whooping cough (pertussis), and to loosen phlegm (as an expectorant). The main components of saffron are crocin, picrocrocin and safranal.

47. Turmeric, Curcuma longa: (rhizome), Manjal, Haldi, Pasupu, Haridra etc names. Turmeric is used in many forms and through many routes of administration, such as – nasal, oral, over the skin etc. Its Sanskrit name indicates its importance. Krimighna – it relieves worm and microbial infection. Peeta/Gauri means has yellow color. Haridra improves skin complexion and cleanses skin. Kanchan means – has color of gold and also brings about golden color to the skin or improves skin glow. Varavarnini- it imparts great color to the skin. Kushtaghna – it helps to eliminate skin diseases. Kandughna – it eliminates itching sensation.

48. Amra Gandhi Haridra, Curcuma Amada: Mango ginger; it is an antibacterial, antifungal, anti-inflammatory and an antioxidant.; used as diuretic, laxative, expectorant, aphrodisiac;

49. Vana haridra, Curcuma aromatica: Karpura Haridra, Kasturi pasupu; It is insecticidal, bactericidal and even anti-carcinogenic too and used routinely in many preparations in India. Haldi containsCurcumin, Curcumenone, Curcone, Curdione, Cineole and others-besides having essential oils.

50. White turmeric, Curcuma zedoaria: C. zerumbet, Kentjur, Zedoary, Kacōramu; the edible rhizome of zedoary has a white interior and a fragrance reminiscent of mango; however, its flavor is more similar to ginger, but differs in taste. It is an antiseptic and a paste applied locally to cuts and wounds helps

healing. The curcumin, epi-pro-curcumenol and many more compounds can be found in Curcuma zedoaria.

51. Jigurudumpa, Curcuma angustifolia: Indian Arrow Root, Thikhur, Thugasheeri, Tvakshira; the rhizomes of C. angustifolia are used to sooth coughs and as such is used to treat bronchitis. Essential oils from the herb have been extracted and are used in antifungal medications. Even these compounds are antibacterial too. The roots of plant are processed to obtain an edible starch (available as tikhur, shotti in market) which has properties similar to arrowroot (Maranta arundinacea, Palagunda) and corn starch. Curcuma angustifolia is also known as East Indian arrowroot.

For extraction of starch, the rhizomes are washed, peeled and kept in sufficient amount of water for overnight. Next these are grinded to get smooth paste. The paste is kept in a vessel and is allowed to settle. Then the excess water lying above the precipitate is drained and the residue is washed by adding water.

This process is repeated to remove all the impurities till pure white starch is obtained which is sun dried to get starch powder. The completely dried starch is stored in bottles for future use.

52. Vanilla, Vanilla planifolia: Vanilla plant is a hybrid of V. planifolia and V. odorata (fruit/beans)–; Vanilla is the second most expensive spice after saffron. An estimated 95% of "vanilla" products are artificially flavoured with vanillin- instead of vanilla fruits. It is labor intensive to purify and mostly used artificial flavoring of bakery products, cakes, ice creams etc.

Fruit extract used primarily as a source of fragrance and as a flavoring agent. The vanilla plant is a source of catechins (also known as polyphenols), which have antioxidant activity and serve as skin-soothing agents.

53. Rasna, Alpinia galanga: Galangal, Thai Ginger, Dumparaashtrakamu, Alpinia galangal, Chinese ginger, Siamese ginger; Siamese ginger (Alpinia galanga) also known as 'Rasna' plant. It is one of four plants known as galangal.

    It is carminative, expectorant, digestive, vulnerary, febrifuge, stimulant, depurative and used in skin diseases, rheumatism, asthma, wounds, fever, hemorrhoids. Lesser galangal, Alpinia officinarum,-both are from ginger family, produced in India, China & many countries; Galangal contains acetoxychavicol acetate, diterpenes, and more compounds. Classical recommendations are for 1 g of the rhizome as a stimulant and carminative.

    Lesser galangal, Alpinia officinarum, is used to treat fever, muscle spasms, intestinal gas, and swelling (inflammation); to kill bacteria; and as a stimulant; related specie with pungent principle due *to* the pungent principle, 5-hydroxy-7-(4-hydroxy- 3-methoxyphenyl)-1-phenyl- 3-heptanone. Lesser galangal, A. speciosa and A. officinarum oils also are effective antifungal agents and are similar as above.

54. Horse radish, Armoracia rusticana: syn. Cochlearia Armorica; Thermogenic, appetizing, digestive, stomachic, laxative, anti- inflammatory, anodyne, refreshing, antibacterial. The roots are antiseptic, aperient, digestive, diuretic, expectorant, rubefacient and stimulant. They should be used in their fresh state. An infusion is used in the treatment of colds, fevers and flu and is of value in the treatment of respiratory and urinary tract infections.

55. Hyssop, Hyssopus officinalis: It is stimulant, carminative & pectoral. It is used in nervous disorders, toothache, pulmonary & uterine troubles. The plant has been used in herbal medicine for the treatment of sore throats, colds, hoarseness, and as an expectorant. Some herbalists also believe that hyssop has beneficial effects for asthma, urinary tract inflammation, and appetite stimulation.

56. Oregano, Origanum vulgare, Sathra, Mariga, Wild marjoram, Madhura vamu:- Stimulant, carminative, stomachic, diuretic, diaphoretic and emmenagogue; The warm infusion releases suppressed menstrual flow. The volatile herb is aromatic, stimulant, rubefacient in rheumatism, toothache & earache. Another is Ajwain ka patta, Thymus vulgaris (leaf). The aromatic thyme plant is a perennial shrub. It is used in bronchitis & whooping cough.

57. Tarragon, Artemisia dracunculus:- Aperient, stomachic, stimulant, febrifuge; The parts of the tarragon plant that grow above the ground are used to make medicine. Tarragon is used to treat digestion problems, poor appetite, water retention, and toothache; to start menstruation; and to promote sleep. In foods and beverages, tarragon is used as a culinary herb.

58. Savory, Satureja hortensis: Antispasmodic, astringent, carminative, laxative, diuretic, stomachic, sudorific, vermifuge; People take summer savory for coughs, sore throat, and intestinal disorders including cramps, indigestion, gas, diarrhea, nausea, and loss of appetite. People with diabetes take it to relieve frequent thirst. It is also used as an aphrodisiac.

Thus, I wish to end my discussion on safe medicinal treatments with conducive herbs and spices- used for generations.

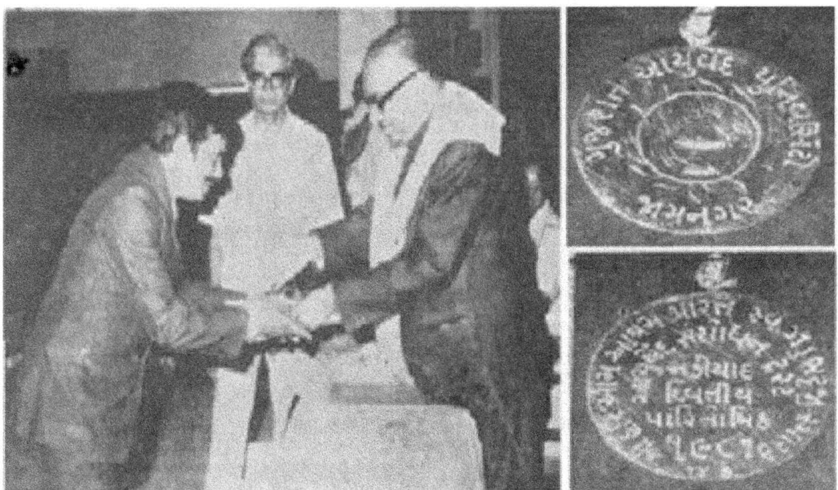

P.G.Rao receiving award for the theory on bioavailability

These are also used for several generations. When one reads the plants collected by Lord Krishna in the sub-merged Dwaraka, one will be surprised to see how old these treatments were known then. There are reported herbs since Ramayan days and there are books published on plants reported in Quran and also in Bible.

Now let us enter into the main herb treatments to tackle more diseases, using medicinal herbs.

6b. Some Complicated Treatments

It is well known that each herb has multisided actions. Hence, whenever a herb is discussed, all its pharmacological uses simultaneously discussed. In home therapy many green leaves, vegetables, spices and other beneficial herbs with their uses discussed.

But, in some treatments, drugs are prepared, processed, even compounded along with some more herbs. With this note, I wish to name few important herbs so that some useful plants can be grown at home.

Many herbs are named after their uses, viz., kushta, mushta, punarnava, anti-asthmatica etc. Charak Samhita is full of such data that cannot be duplicated here. So, hardened diseases need stronger doses herbs which need ayurvedic physicians' guidance.

Where to start the discussion?

the answer begins with the body cleaners.

6.v.a. The Body Cleaners

They consist of demulcents, laxatives, diuretics, purgatives, GIT cleaners, worm killers/expellers- all act in different levels.

Any substance that relieves irritation of the mucous membranes in the mouth or a substance that relieve inflammation or irritation is a demulcent. Laxative is a medicine, food or drink that somebody can take to make his/her get rid of solid waste from the body easily.

Diuretics help the body get rid of extra fluid and salt. They are useful to treat high blood pressure, edema etc. The present discussion is thus a continuation of the home therapy treatments.

Some examples are Liquorice (Glycyrrhiza glabra), Corn Silk (Zea mays), Flaxseed (Linum usitatissimum), Lungwort (Sticta pulmonaria), Isabgol/Plantago ovata (Psyllium), (In home therapy some herbs are already covered). More details are below:

a. i. Isabgol/Plantago ovata (Psyllium seed husk): It is an herb that is native to Asia, the Mediterranean region and North Africa. Known as a common remedy for effective weight loss and clearing.

a. ii. Goksura or Palleru fruit is cooling, diuretic, tonic, aphrodisiac, urinary diseases treat calculus, gout, kidney and even impotence. Goksura, Tribulus terrestris, Palleru, Caltrops, Puncture vine,

Trikantaka, Chotagokhru- are different names. The fruit cooling, diuretic, tonic, aphrodisiac, urinary diseases treat calculus, gout, kidney and even impotence. Gokshura is mostly recommended for male health including virility and vitality and specifically more catered towards cardiovascular and uro-genital health. It is supposed to possess testosterone boosting properties. Given a 60% saponin extract, a dose of between 200-450mg a day or 1-3 gm fruits grinded and boiled.

a. iii. Musab-bar, Aloe vera/A. barbadensis, Aloe, Kalabanda, Elavaluka, Ghirta-kumari, Kumari, etc. names. The use of aloe extract increases bladder capacity to hold urine, yet gives time-hence, named "musa-saber or musabbar". Useful in diabetes, wounds, stomachic,

purgative, emmenagogue, contain aloin, a polysaccharide and anthracene derivative. Aloe has blood thinning action. It is very useful against cholesterol. Because of its mild laxative action and wound healing properties, regular intake of mild doses of aloe vera in the form of capsule or juice, is very beneficial. It is stomachic, emmenagogue, purgative, and anthelmintic.

The root used in colic and, contains arabino-glucan- polymers and anthraquinone derivatives. Aloe indica or Aloe vera is synonym to above.

a.iv. Yarrow, Achillea millefolium, commonly known as yarrow is a flowering plant, native to Europe, yet located in India too. Yarrow tea contains flavonoids and alkaloids that may relieve symptoms of depression and anxiety. Yarrow has long been used to treat digestive ulcers, injuries and cures even irritable bowels. IBS or irritable bowel syndrome has symptoms of stomach pain, diarrhea, bloating, and constipation. In fact, this herb contains several flavonoids and alkaloids, which are plant compounds known to relieve digestive complaints. Yarrow is also used for fever, common cold, hay fever, absence of menstruation, dysentery, diarrhea, loss of appetite, gastro-intestinal irritation.

a. v. St. John's wort or Klamath weed or Hypericum perforatum commonly known as Saint-John's-wort. This genus is of nearly 500 species – an invasive, noxious-weeds. It is used to treat bruises and burns also. Its berries are *poisonous* and so, should not be ingested. Consumption can cause photosensitization. St- Johns-wort flowers in a large retro mug to get a healthy tea.

6. a2. Purgatives: In nutshell, list of Purgative or cathartic or laxative-s can be Croton Tiglium > Ricinus communis, Cuscuta reflexa, Turpeth/Ipomoea turpethum, Ipomoea hederacea,- besides common use herbs like munaga, senna, rhubarb, aloe etc. They become lighter in descending order. But let us begin with some lighter versions.

a. vi. Drumstick, Moringa oleifera, munaga; It has important minerals, and is a good source of protein, vitamins, β-carotene, amino acids & various phenolic compounds. Its fruits look like sticks used for beating stomach used as a vegetable; Its root is stimulant, and used in paralytic affections, intermittent fevers and a cardiac tonic too. It can also be used for epilepsy treatment, useful in fainting and giddiness, nervous debility and bowel affections. Its bark is abortifacient and flowers are aphrodisiac. The seed oil is used externally for rheumatism also. It is also used in wound healing.

a. vii. Some plants like cassia are known body cleansers. Aragvadha, Cassia fistula, Akkotu, Suvarnaka, Amaltas Kritamala, Rela chettu, Golden Shower, Indian-Laburnum, Pudding Pipe Tree, purging cassia, Indian laburnum: root, bark, seed, leaf- purgative; contains xanthone glycosides and also 2% anthraquinones, 24% crude protein, and 50% carbohydrates; The various parts of the tree like the bark, root, flowers, leaves, fruit pulp are used medicinally and have several health benefits. The pulp obtained from the fruit is called the cassia pulp and is known to be an effective laxative and used for constipation. It is a safe drug can be consumed by all. Its root is a tonic that helps in reducing fevers, while leaves and stem are useful in treating intestinal disorders too.

Indian senna, Cassia absus, Chaksu; the plant is a small herb growing up to 50 cm bearing reddish yellow flowers. The seeds are black. Chakshushya is known senna. Cassia angustifolia, or senna is also known as Cassia absus. Chaksu seeds have many uses making it one of the most sought after ayurveda that can be used in the form of decoction, powder and even juice. Chaksu Seeds used for Lowering Blood Pressure.

Used externally as a paste or collyrium in eye diseases like conjunctivitis (Netra abishyanda) Its roots contain Chaksine. Chaksine is found to be antibacterial. It stimulates contraction of plain muscles like uterus, intestine, bladder and muscles in the blood vessels. Chaksine has ganglion blocking property. Seed contain Beta Sitosterol, Hydnocarpin, and Apigenin & Raffinose. Its leaves contain Quercetin and Rutin.

Sonamukhi, Cassia angustifolia, Alexandrian senna, Senna Alexandrina, Swarna Patri; It is used as a laxative, contains hydroxy anthracene glycosides, also known as Senna Sennoside. These glycosides stimulate the peristalsis of the colon and alter colonic absorption and secretion resulting in fluid accumulation and expulsion. The leaves of this herb are made into a tea and marketed as a weight-loss aid under the brand name Slim-Mate.

True senna, Kaseya, Nelatangedu; Cassia acutifolia, Cassia angustifolia, Cassia lanceolata, Cassia senna – all are similar. Senna is a powerful cathartic used in the treatment of constipation, working through a stimulation of intestinal peristalsis. Senna is mainly for treating a fever or for clearing Pitta from the small intestines. The leaves were sometimes made into a paste and applied to various skin diseases. Ringworm and acne were both treated in this way. Its leaves and fruits laxative, purgative that produce side effects like diarrhea, nausea, and dehydration, if improperly used. It contains Kaempferol and other compounds including anthraquinone derivatives.

Dadrumurdan, Cassia alata, Guajava, Candle bush, Simayakatti, Ringworm shrub, Seemaiagathi; Guajava is a beautiful flowering shrub, produces pretty yellow flowers in a column that resemble the yellow candlesticks, thus named candle bush. Also used for killing ring worms and for cleaning ulcers. Apply the leaves grinded in coconut oil and apply on the skin thrice a day. The leaf extracts cure asthma, fungal infections and eczema. Taken seeds flowers, leaves as extracts to rebuke stomach problems, but, not good in pregnancy.

Tanged, Cassia auriculata, Avaram, Tanner's Cassia, Tarwad; Senna auriculata is a legume tree, commonly avaram senna. The flower, leaves, stem, root, and unripe fruit are used for treatment, especially in Ayurvedic medicine. Its leaves can be used as anti-oxidant, asthma, astringent, in diabetes, eye infections (conjunctivitis), joint and muscle pain (rheumatism), constipation, jaundice, liver disease, and urinary tract disorders. The root used for skin diseases and seeds as anti-diabetic and leaves & fruits as anthelmintic.

Kasmarda, Cassia occidentalis, Negro coffee, Kasivinda, Coffee weed, Kasundi, Tanged, Kasintha, Kolla- dalasari- aku, Pedda tagarisa; Kasamarda is used as an aphrodisiac, improves digestion, cleanses throat, useful in cough, balance all the three Doshas etc. Its leaves are considered poisonous. It is used for the treatment of cough, cold, eczema, dyspepsia and also filariasis. Cassia seeds are a good herbal treatment for lowering the blood pressure. The leaves and pods (shells) are usually administered in the Ayurvedic and Unani systems as infusion- as a tonic in low doses. Coffee out of Senna seeds are attributed with blood purifying and diuretic properties. The herb has been traditionally used to normalize bowel movements.

Purging Cassia, Cassia senna, Cassia lanceolata, Bhupadma, Bhumiari, Pitapushpi, Swarnamukhi, swarnapatrika, Tinnevelly senna, Senna nela-tangedu; Another is sickle-pod, Senna obtusifolia or Chinese senna, – it is also similar. The leaves and the fruit of the plant are used to make medicine. It is used to treat constipation and also to clear the bowel before diagnostic tests such as colonoscopy. Senna is also used for irritable bowel syndrome (IBS), hemorrhoids, and weight loss. Senna is known to deplete potassium, and sodium as being diuretic. So, senna may cause diarrhea, caution is warranted in patients receiving warfarin, because diarrhea can reduce the absorption of vitamin K and increase the risk of bleeding. The drug consists of nearly dried and ripe pods.

Kolkasunda, Cassia sophera, Kasmarda, Kasivinda, Algarrobilla, Kasunda, Baner, Kasaundi; The plant is credited with the same properties as C. occidentalis. In Bangladesh, root juice used for fevers and as diuretic; paste from leaves used for ringworm and sores. Boil 5-7 gm of dried Cassia sophera with the same amount of mint in two cups of water until the water is reduced to a half. It has yellow flowers in corymbose racemes. Senna sophera was formerly called Cassia sophera. Its decoction is used in acute bronchitis and acts on respiratory system as an expectorant and bronchodilator. It acts on GIT as anthelminthic and cathartic. Its mother tincture is prepared from the roots and also acts on the skin as antiseptic. It contains active principle emodin and also chrysophanic acid. It is a medicine of bronchial asthma in children below 12 years of age.

Chakra Marda, Cassia Tora, Tagarisa, Sickle senna, Sickle pod, Tora, Coffee pod, Tovar, Chakvad, Prapanna, Fetid cassia; Different parts of the plant (Leaves, seed, and root) are reputed for their medicinal value. It is well recognized traditional medicine as laxative and is useful for treatment of leprosy, ringworm infection, ophthalmic, skin diseases and liver disorders. Several chemical compounds such as Anthraquinone glycosides, Flavonoids, Naphthopyrone glycosides, Phenolic compounds, etc. have been isolated from this plant. The leaf decoctions made of one-part leaves and ten parts waters, given to children as two ounces to cure fevers during teething. The leaves are very nutritious and tasty when cooked. Seeds, roots and leaves as poultice used to cure skin diseases and even leprosy. Seeds used as coffee in some parts of Africa.

Many more species of cassia do exist and almost all cassia species in general are safe for internal consumption as medicine, with varying laxative properties. But check literature before use.

a. viii. Another good gene is Sida species; Bon-methi, Nagabala, Sida spinosa, Gulsakari, Mayir-manijjam, Prickly sida; it is found throughout the hotter parts of India and Sri Lanka. Its root & bark are used in irritability of bladder as a decoction. Its roots are tonic & diaphoretic and as extract given in debility and fevers. All Sida species have similar properties and hence are put together. Kuruntotti, Sida alnifolia, Palampadu; its leaves, flower, fruit are used even for its fragrancy. Its parts leaves, flower, fruit and roots are used in medicine and used in the treatment of fever, hypertension, hernia and oedema. Sida alnifolia contained ephedrine, in highest in Sida (0.92%).

Arrow leaf sida, Atibala, Sida rhombifolia, Tenacham; It has significant medicinal uses for which it is cultivated in India. The pounded leaves are used to relieve swelling, the fruits are used to relieve headache, the mucilage is used as an emollient, and the root is used to treat rheumatism. Its roots contain traces of ephedrine alkaloids in low percentage. Choose one out of choice.

Janglimethi, Sida acuta, S. carpinifolia: Horn bean-leaved sida, Bala, Visa-boddi; the root of sida acuta is used as stomachic, diaphoretic, and anti-pyretic. It is regarded as astringent, cooling, tonic, useful in nervous and urinary diseases. It is used in blood disorders and bile formation. It has an alkaloid, cryptolepine, responsible for anti-spasmodic activity. The decoction of the plant is taken orally to cure urinary diseases and impotency. It contains phenolics, ferulic acid etc., Bon-methi, Nagabala, Sida spinosa, Gulsakari, Mayir-manijjam, Prickly sida; it is found throughout the hotter parts of India and Sri Lanka. Its root & bark are used in irritability of bladder as a decoction. Its roots are tonic & diaphoretic and as extract given in debility and fevers. All Sida species have similar properties and hence are put together.

Kuruntotti, Sida alnifolia, Palampadu; its leaves, flower, fruit are used even for its fragrancy. Its leaves, flower, fruit and roots are used in medicine and used in the treatment of fever, hypertension, hernia and oedema. Sida alnifolia contained ephedrine, in highest in Sida (0.92%).

Arrow leaf sida, Atibala, Sida rhombifolia, Tenacham; It has significant medicinal uses for which it is cultivated in India. The pounded leaves are used to relieve swelling, the fruits are used to relieve headache, the mucilage is used as an emollient, and the root is used to treat rheumatism. Its roots contain traces of ephedrine alkaloids in low percentage.

Janglimethi, Sida acuta, S. carpinifolia: Horn bean-leaved sida, Bala, Visa-boddi; the root of sida acuta is used as stomachic, diaphoretic, and anti-pyretic. It is regarded as astringent, cooling, tonic, useful in nervous and urinary diseases. It is used in blood disorders and bile formation. It has an alkaloid, cryptolepine, responsible for anti-spasmodic activity. The decoction of the plant is taken orally to cure urinary diseases and impotency. It contains phenolics, ferulic acid etc.,

Choose one cassia specie out of multiple choice mentioned above for use-which suits you.

a.ix. Cuscuta reflexa is a parasitic weed plant;- used for urination, jaundice, muscle pain and coughs; treatment of body pains and itchy skin.

a.x. My late mother used to administer castor oil to me every month. This is how through the customs/traditions, the people have maintained better health. Arandi, leaves are applied as poultice, cure headache; seed purgative, fish poison; seed oil, root, leaf-used as purgative contain ricinine & others ricinolein, even its acid along with stearic, linoleic, palmitic acids, sitosterol, squalene etc.

Now-a day's liquid paraffin 50 ml can also do the job well. Now liquid paraffin is used along with milk of magnesia-called cremaffin-forte for slow emptying or dulcoflex for faster elimination. But let us begin with some lighter versions.

6.v.bi. Vermifuge/worm expellers: As anthelmintic, daruhaldi or Berberis, is the best/safest and widely used even in few liver tonics;

As worm expeller, Turmeric raw root is burnt and mixed with castor oil and given even to children. It expels within 12hrs. Alternatively, Areca catechu, Carica papaya seeds, Punica granatum, Mehndi, Melilotus Philippines's, Embelia ribes, etc., are reputed vermifuges.

ii. Worm infestation: Use either (a)vayu-vidanga seeds or (b)seeds of mehndi- grinded to paste and consumed with some honey or (c) consume munaga tree delicate shoots-direct early morning or take as (rasam) tamarind plus salt & leaves boiled extract.

b. iii. Warts, gout, rheumatism: Hirantutiya, Colchicum luteum – to cure warts, gout, rheumatism, and diseases of liver and spleen; It commonly find use as a carminative, laxative, & an aphrodisiac with colchicine @0.25%. Gloriosa superba- is another herb with higher % of colchicines, identified with thanks to advancements in chemistry.

a. Vayu-vidangalu, Embelia ribes, Vidanga or Vaivrang or Janntughna, Kapala, Chitratandula, and Krmighna: Its fruits, seeds, roots and even its leaves are used as medicine. It is used to kill all types of bacteria, virus and fungus. Dried fruit anthelmintic, astringent, used in scorpion bite, Vidanga is best herb used for worm infestation that includes roundworm, threadworm and tapeworms. This herb is also very effective for infants that are suffering with worm infestation. Contain @5% embelin a hydroxyl quinone derivative, along with quercitol and fatty ingredients & clears chest troubles.

b.b. Vauding', Embelia tsjeriam- cottam, 'Vidanga'; It is a plant- commonly harvested from the wild for local use. Its medicinal properties are not proven. Vidanga is one of the powerful anti-parasitic herbs of Ayurveda. Both fruits are used against ringworm and skin diseases, fruits for external application and seeds for internal use.

b.c. Kamala, Melilotus Philippines's, Monkey-face Tree, Kapila, Sinduri, Kumkum tree, Red Berry tree; the fruits are with glands and hair on it. Kumkum, glands and hair on the fruit-bitter, anthelmintic, cathartic, used for deworming in cattle. Contains mainly phenols, diterpenoids, steroids, flavonoids etc. Kamala acts quickly as a purgative in humans too, and often causes much griping and nausea, but seldom causes vomiting. It may be given in water mucilage or syrup; the worm is usually expelled at the third or fourth stool; if it fails to act, the dose is repeated after four hours. Kamala is insoluble in cold water or boiling water.

The resin is the most active constituent, and is dissolved by ether, chloroform, alcohol. Its fruit contains resin @ 78%. The bark of kamala is also an excellent antimicrobial agent. *The* root of the tree is used in dyeing, and for cutaneous eruptions, also used by the Arabs internally for leprosy and in solution to remove freckles and pustules.

b.d. Dhumrapatra, Aristolochia bracteata, Esvaraveru, Aduthina-palai, Aristolochia, Pipevine, Dutchman's pipe; it is known as a "worm killer"; Its members are commonly known as birthwort, and are widespread and occur in the most diverse climates. plant

purgative, anthelmintic, emetic, leaves as juice applied on ulcers, paste of leaves mixed with castor oil on eczema in even children, decoction of root for expelling round worms;

b.e. Most powerful purgative is Jamalgota (Croton Tiglium), also called Purging Croton, which has stimulant action on bowel movement. It has potent side effects, which result in cramps causing defecation and loose stools. Colchicine containing are toxic. Use them with physician's supervision.

6.v.c. Anti-diarrheal/febrifuge, is needed. The best anti-diarrheal is curd. Even, pomegranate, or soap-nut extract are also anti-diarrheal. There are many herbs that are wormicidal and thus anti-diarrheal. But if the problem is severe, then consult Genus Holarrhena or Cosnium or Berberis.

c. i. Indian Barberry, Berberis aristata, Berberis vulgaris, Daruharidra, Chitra, Darhald, Daruhaldi, Darurajani, Darvi amberparisi, Indian Lyceum; Daruhaldi is used to treat liver, ulcers, fever, intestinal infection, cuts, eye and skin diseases and also most common use as antidiarrheal.

Rasaut is prepared by boiling roots and lower parts of the stem of daruhaldi with sixteen times their weight of water and cooked to one fourth level then filtered hot and again the filtrate is concentrated to get thick gum. This when gets dried becomes rasaut. It is de-obstruent, used in jaundice, eye infections, and also antidiarrheal. Rasaut is used to cure stomach infection, piles, ulcers, fever and constipation also. It is rich in berberine type alkaloids. It is rich in berberine 2-2.5% alkaloids; seco-bis-benzil-isoquinoline or simple isoquinoline alkaloids; Daruharidra, Berberis asiatica, Indian Barberry, Chutro, Rasanjan, marpyashi, Tree Turmeric, Chitra; other sources of rasaut are B. lyceum, B. aristata, B. nepalensis, B. vulgaris; The roots are used in treating ulcers, urethral discharges, ophthalmia, jaundice, fevers etc. The roots contain 2.1% and the stems 1.3% berberine. It is taken internally to treat fevers and is used externally to treat conjunctivitis and other inflammations of the eyes. It is mostly used as a cure dysentery and liver tonic. Its properties are similar to B. aristata.

c.ii. Manupasupu, Cosnium fenestratum, Daruharidra, Daru haridra, Jhar-i-haldi, Mara Munjal, Tree Turmeric; its stem is also having anti-oxidants, that are found to be useful in diabetes. This is the tree turmeric – also available in warmer climates with berberine @1-3% ext. Its bark and root bitter, tonic, used in intestinal fevers, The root bark contains berberine, quaternary ammonium salt of isoquinoline alkaloids with antibacterial, antifungal, antiviral and antioxidant, anti-inflammatory, anti-tumor and anti-diabetic activities.

It is known for quick wound healing, useful in diabetes and urinary tract diseases, It is also useful in the treatment of pain and itching related disorders related to eyes, ears and oral cavity, & anti-inflammatory and relieves skin diseases with itching. Used in snake bite, extract of root bark bitter and tonic & also used in intestinal fevers.

c.iii. Goldenseal, Hydrastis Canadensis, Yellow Indian paint, Eye root, Ground raspberry, Indian dye, Jaundice root, orange root; it also contains isoquinoline alkaloids such as berberine (2.5%) & hydrastine (1.5 – 4%), hence anti-diarrheal; Contains hydrastine and berberine. It is nutritive system and also with the circulatory system. This is anti-diarrheal and also used to treat arrow wounds & ulcers. It is documented to be a uterine stimulant. It extracts in diluted amounts used as eye wash. Large doses cause nausea, anxiety, depression, seizures and paralysis also.

c.iv. Indrajao, Holarrhena antidysenterica, Pink-eyed cerbera, Girimallika, Kodise-pala-tiga, Pum Kutaja, Kurchi, Conessi bark, Veppalai, palakondsa; it is antidiarrheal. Used for treatment of constipation, colic, fevers, and diarrhea; seed used as febrifuge & worm killer; bark used in dysentery, dried powder rubbed over the body for dropsy; seeds astringent, febrifuge, fever, dysentery, diarrhea, & intestinal worms; contain conessine, Kur-chine & kur-chicine. It is the best medicine for amoebiasis.

6.vi.d. Next is digestives and jaundice curers:

Liver: Indigestion can be due to liver dysfunction. Coming to general health, liver is a vital organ that digests most food particles and always needs to be functional like heart, and brain and body has no substitute to these organs in the body. Here, hydrotherapy or home cure treats in easing the liver. If leafy vegetables are consumed frequently, jaundice may not reach a person at all.

Hence, if liver is treated in the initial levels, many diseases may not sustain in our body, thus making the liver treatment important. If the liver is either sick or struck with jaundice (kamala or pasiri) what is a possible remedy in the modern medicine? Then only few vitamins are the suggested medicines along with sugarcane juice as a staple and sustainable diet.

In case of a troubled liver or stomachache or fever- in ayurveda-fasting is an established mode of correction. In the modern medicine too, ornithine tablets activate the sluggish liver. In AP, the fever recovery is done with curry leaves (Murraya koengii – rich in free amino acids) and light spice like jeera, chili and haldi- adds taste too.

But jaundice needs naturally additional treatments. There are more than seventy liver extracts containing herbal extracts to treat liver troubles-as reported in Indian herbal pharmacopoeia. These extracts vary from region to region.

6.vii.d. Liver tonics: About seventy liver related herbal tonics were looked in India for their contents.

d.i. Out of which, there are 28 liver tonics (preparations) that contain kalmegh. It is used even now for treating jaundice.

d.ii. The drug kutki or katuki or katukarohini (Picrorrhiza Kurroa) if taken in hand & broken into two pieces, one finds black scar in the center of the root. This drug is present in @10 tonics.

d.iii. Another is Tal makhana (Astercantha longifolia) is used in ten preparations. Its seeds @10 gm. if soaked in hot water, left overnight & drunk in the morning, gives support to the ligaments (joint).

d.iv. Later comes vidanga, (Embelia ribes), 8 preparations, celery, (Apium graveolens)-8 preparations, giloe or giloy (Tinospora Cordifolia) – 8 preparations, and ajowan

(Trachyspermum Ammi), 8 preparations. Further even Bhumya-malaki (Phyllanthus niruri), mulhathi (Glycyrrhiza glabra), kasni (Cichorium intybus), papaya (Carica papaya), and daruharidra (Berberis aristata), are also present in some selected liver extracts.

d.v. Milk thistle (Silybum marianum), also helps to prevent the depletion of glutathione, with antioxidant activity and is believed to be ten times more potent than Vitamins.

d.vi. In some places Bhumyamalaki (Phyllanthus niruri) is the preferred drug for treatment of liver/jaundice.

vii. Turmeric-root (Curcuma longa), is anti-inflammatory and antioxidant, the polyphenols are also shown to be beneficial in reducing the risk of fatty liver disease caused by stress.

d. viii. Dandelion (Taraxacum officinale) root aids liver function by improving the body's ability to remove toxins while also boosting the production of bile. A Korean study its root helped to prevent damage to the liver caused by environmental toxins such as alcohol and chemicals.

d.ix. The next best herb is pigweed or punarnava (Boerhaavia diffusa) – present in more than a dozen liver tonics. Even sunthi (ginger) is known to preserve liver health.

x. A root vegetable beet-root (Beta vulgaris) is not only an excellent source of fiber but also folic acid, manganese, and potassium. Beet-root contains important antioxidant compounds such as beta lain pigments which have been found to scavenge free radicals and reduce inflammation throughout the body.

d.xi. In addition, inorganic elements like magnesium, manganese, molybdenum and even selenium have numerous health benefits.

The list can further extend to Aloe barbadensis fresh leaf juice, Azadirachta indica/neem leaf or ext.; roots or stem ext.; Carica papaya leaf ext. or male flower ext. or unripe fruit; Cassia fistula leaf ext. or fresh fruit pulp ext.; Cassia occidentalis leaf or ext.; Centella asiatica aerial parts or leaf; Euphorbia hirta aerial parts; Lawsonia inermis leaf or bark; Melia azedarach leaf for pain in liver; Ocimum Americanum twig for jaundice; Plumbago zeylanica roots or ext.; Ricinus communis root or seed aq. Ext; Rubia cordifolia root; Tribulus terristris fruits ext.; Tridax procumbens whole plant; Psidium guajava leaf ext. or fruit ext.

These are some examples for curing the liver disfunction like using roasted powder of Curry leaves. Probably it can be the reason that one finds these leaves in most south Indian cookery. In fact, a vast majority of diseases are cured through liver tonics. This list accounts for the most reputed herbs in liver tonics.

6.viii.e. Suggested tonics:

Some examples of the suggested treatment given-that were unreported or combinations suggested by my friend & late colleague, Dr. V. N. Gupta – a pharmacist.

Neem or Azadirachta indica – its leaves dried and powdered, @ 6-12 gm. with honey- consumed daily for @ one week.

Another is Guduchi or Tinospora cordifolia – its fresh stem or delicate bark crushed through expeller or crushed and squeezed to get juice, its juice @12 gm. is mixed with honey 12 gm. for 1 week.

The next is Daruharidra or Berberis aristata – whole plant (bark powder or bark extract called rasaut)) powder-1 to 3 gm. taken with honey daily twice a day (BDS)- most suited for Assam region.

A mixture of punarnava or Boerhaavia diffusa or tella galejeru or also known as pigweed- well powdered, mixed with equal quantity of three myrobalans (Terminalia arjuna, T. bellerica, T. chebula in equal proportions) – the mixture treated with sterile luke- warm water (1:4 as w/v) stirred and squeezed, liquid 6-12 gm. with honey thrice a day.

If jaundice crisis is severe, stems of Tinospora cordifolia, fresh leaves of Adhatoda vasica, Picrorrhiza kurroa whole herb fresh/ dried, fresh leaves of Azadirachta indica, Swertia chirata and three myrobalans mixture- and a fresh aq. extract is drawn (as 1:4 w/v) & concentrated to get thick syrup. Take this syrup 6-12 ml and mixed with honey (1:1) and taken as 6-12 ml BDS for five days. It can go up to 30 ml daily if severe. Such extracts can be stored as tablets or a goli or as syrup upon dilution with honey, glycerol and boiled water.

It is Kalmegh, (Andrographis paniculata),- present in more than 20 liver tonics in India & used for liver complaints including jaundice. But, one of the best liver tonics is gallic acid, present in many species of Terminalia, like haritaki or vibhitaki. There are other liver stimulants like Boerhaavia diffusa, Picrorrhiza kurroa, Solanum nigrum or brihati etc.-more details given with liver.

e.i. Kalmegh, Andrographis paniculata: green Chiretta, Kirata tikta, Bhunimba or Kirataa or Kirayat or Nelavemu-or Nilavemu or Nelavepu; It is- used for centuries in treating ulcer, contains andrographolide (0.8- 2.5%) responsible for the action.

It is also used to treat leprosy, bronchitis, skin diseases, flatulence, diabetes, high blood pressure, colic, influenza, dysentery, dyspepsia and even malaria; Kalmegh has been used for liver complaints including jaundice, fever, act as an anti-inflammatory and immuno-stimulant.

Andrographis extract has been studied for use as an immunostimulant in upper respiratory tract infections. Extracts of Andrographis have demonstrated hypoglycemic action.

e.ii. Bhuiamla: Phyllanthus niruri, Bhunimba or Nela usiri; plant diuretic, dropsical affections; contain phyllanthin, a bitter substance, but has no quinine, yet used in malaria, cures jaundice or all liver affections.

It is used as a folk medicine for treating kidney stones, gallbladder stones, liver related diseases such as liver cancer & jaundice, apart from these it is also administered for diuretic, hypoglycemic and hypertension cases and it also shows anti-inflammatory, anti-tumor, and antinociceptive.

e. iii. Kutki, Picrorrhiza kurroa: Katuka Rohini, Kuru; Akutam, katuki; Picrorrhiza kurroa is a powerful Ayurvedic herb used in treating mainly chronic fever, skin disorders and diabetes. It is also used in purgation (Virechana in Panchakarma) procedure. It is used as cathartic, stomachic, used in fever, dyspepsia and purgative. It has been traditionally used to treat upper respiratory tract and reduce fevers.

It also cures jaundice and acute viral hepatitis also. It cures chronic fevers and skin diseases. It contains kutkin 3.4%, the bitter principle, responsible for many pharmacological actions and used in a dozen liver tonics.

e.iv. Punarnava, Boerhaavia diffusa, Pigweed, Tella-galijeru: Punarnava repairs the abnormalities or injured parts. Punarnava has two varieties, white, Sweta punarnava and red, rakta punarnava, both useful as above; white is rich and as tannins red is rich. Ayurvedics use red often as no confusion with specie punarnavi (Trianthema monogyna) which is also useful and edible. Red punarnava is considered to be anti-diabetic and diuretic – as it repairs the worn-out parts. In different places has also been used for pain relief, anti-inflammation, jaundice, and treating indigestion.

e.v. Gallic acid and ellagic acids are liver tonics. Thus, Vibhitaki haritaki, & pashanbhed are also automatic liver stimulants

e.vi. Pashanbhed, Bergenia ligulata, Pig Squeak, Pakhanabheda, Patharcua, Bergenia Ciliata, Saxifraga ligulata; This plant has been recognized for dissolving kidney stones & bladder stones and also useful in fevers. It is diuretic, anti-diabetic, wound healer, astringent, cardiotonic, expectorant, hepatoprotective, antipyretic, anti-cancer and antiprotozoal properties.

It contains bergenin, tannic acid, gallic acid, stigmasterol, arbutin, caryophyllene, eudesmol and asarone. Its extract is applied on boils and ophthalmia. Probably, Gallic and ellagic acids are helping in digestion of stones along with other tannins.

Genus- Terminalia & Solanum provide several plants for this purpose- besides many other uses.

6.ix.f. Now, let us look for a speech stimulator. It is here coming sweet flag, Acorus

calamus, Haimavati, "bhutanashini", Bach, Vacha (vacha means talk), vasambu, Vaca: it is Thermogenic, constipating, emmenagogue, intellect promoting, emetic, carminative, tranquilizing, resuscitative, expectorant, stomachic, sedative, sudorific, antipyretic, nervine tonic.

Crush Vaca and boil it in water. Boil till the water is reduced to half quantity. Filter and drink the boiled water. For babies and infants show vasa directly on flame till it is burnt and become black. Use a tong or pot holder to heat on direct flame. Now grind the burnt root and store the powder in an air tight container.

Some people coat the vasa with castor oil before showing it on fire. It can be mixed with honey to consume it. Improves speech, intelligence and also it induces contractions in uterus. Bach or vasa is used as emetic, stomachic, as nervine tonic and anti-dysenteric in children. It contains acoradin, 2,4,5-trimethoxy benzaldehyde, 2,5-dimethoxy- benzoquinone, spathulenol, calamendiol, galangin, and sitosterol. 6.X.G. How to eliminate a throat/chest problem? The best throat and lung cleaner is garlic. It is a natural herbal remedy for chest congestion and sore throat. It has anti-inflammatory and antiviral properties. Some more are tulasi with 85% eugenol in it, mulethi, giloy, sonth, cinnamon, etc., all covered in spices.

i. Mul-Hathi, Glycyrrhiza glabra, (Yastimadhu, Madhuka, Liquorice, lico-rice, Mulatti, Atimadhuram); Mul Hathi or meaning root eliminated. It is given as a max. dose per day is 3 grams- thrice a day- for colic gastritis, stomach ulcers, useful in inflammation, cough and cold; tonic, laxative, digestive, demulcent, Genito-urinary diseases, bronchitis, sore throat, and scorpion sting. It is the most familiar herb and used as a flavoring in foods, beverages, and tobacco. The creeper's root bark- or licorice is the medicine. Glycyrrhizin (glycyrrhizic acid) constitutes 10 – 25% of root extract. Its saponin is comprised of a triterpenoid aglycone – along with many other compounds.

g.ii. Giloy: Somida, Tinospora cordifolia is a herbaceous vine indigenous to the Indian subcontinent. It has been used in Ayurveda to treat various disorders, but there is no clinical evidence for the effectiveness of such treatment. Amrita, guduchi means something that protects the whole body. Giloy is used in chronic fever, improves respiration & also immunity, improve digestion, reduces stress and anxiety, helps in the treatment arthritis and gout etc., uses.

g.iii. If cough also gets attached, it can turn towards asthma, then: At this level also, mul-hathi works, but better is trikatu-made-up of three spices, maricha, maga and ginger- known as vata-pitta-kapha haratvam (eliminates every trouble). It is maricha that brought awards to our group. Ginger dissolves every digestive trouble of stomach.

Maricha as a powder with jaggery, made into a goli and chewed to eliminate cough. Still better is medicine being vasaka (Glyodin-terp-vasaka- is a well-known syrup with probably glycerin). Cough is also treated with vibhitaki chewing. Its compounds are also liver tonics.

g.iv. Asthma/tubercolosis: here the remedy is vibhitaki chew is good. But if cough and asthma, a bronchodilator like vasaka needed. If it takes serious turn, it can tend to be tubercular,-answer is antamul.

g.v. Brenkhad, Adhatoda vasica, Justicia adhatoda, Adusa, Malabar nut, Adulsa, Addasaramu, Adamkabu, Adampaka, Vasaka, Pavettai; vasaka- wp-cures asthma, rheumatism, insecticidal; flowers, leaves, roots antiseptic; leaves and roots in chronic bronchitis; its leaves, flowers and bark are used in medicine. The fresh leaves of vasica are chewed, sometimes with ginger, because of their stimulant effect on the respiratory system. It is an antispasmodic and expectorant, and has been used for centuries with much success to treat asthma, chronic bronchitis, and other respiratory conditions. It contains prominent quinazoline alkaloids known as vasicine and vasicinone in the leaves and its roots contain the alkaloids l-vasicinone, deoxy-vasicine, vasicinol etc.

g.vi. Harmal, Peganum harmala, Seemagorita vittulu, Esfand, Wild rue, Syrian rue; Its whole plant extract is aphrodisiac, emmenagogue and abortifacient. Its seeds are narcotic and given in fevers & used as remedy for tapeworm. The root ext. kills lice and decoction of leaves used in rheumatism. It contains alkaloids harmine, harmaline and peganine (vasicine). It is peganine and vasicinone are bronchodilators.

g.vii. Antamul, Tylophora indica or Tylophora asthmatica, Indian Ipecac, Vallippula, Vettipala; Antomula means ends the root of asthma (leaves). It has known to possess anti-inflammatory activities against asthma, bronchitis, bronchial asthma, tuberculosis, and rheumatism; Antamul is medicinal perennial vine which is found in eastern, central and southern India. This plant is like ipecuanha, with its leaves emetic, diaphoretic & expectorant. Tylophora is useful in countering asthma and allergy. It is an antipyretic and diuretic it contains tylophorine in 0.44% on dry weight basis. For treating tuberculosis, it is given in combination with mercury complexes for recovery.

6.xi.h. One needs killers of infections/worms/bacilli. The best drug is trikatu. It is a mixture of Maricha, Maga and ginger- known vata-pitta and kapha haratvam (eliminate every type). It is maricha that was proven to be a bioavailability enhancer by my group (see back pages- spices). Here comes preventer of infections, gorinta.

h. i. Gorinta, Lawsonia inermis: (goru – inta means protected nails) Henna, Mehndi, Madayantika, Mendiga, gorinta-are different names. It is a remedy against almost any disease and its seeds serve like lead-wort seeds, but of lesser potency. bark jaundice cure, enlargement of spleen, also skin; leaf decoction used in sore throat, flowers refrigerant; leaf sugar is remedy for spermatorrhea.

Its bark extract cures jaundice, enlargement of spleen and also cure skin diseases. Its leaf decoction cures sore throat and flowers refrigerant. Its leaf if consumed with sugar is remedy for spermatorrhea. Its leaf powder or its paste used for staining nails, hair and even beard. The plant has a wide range of Phyto-chemicals which include lawsone, isoplumbagin, lawsoniaside, syringinoside, agrimonolide and others.

It is safe and can be grown at home. It contains iso-plumbagin in low concentrations in its seeds. Its brothers, plumbagin rich plants, known as chitrak or leadwort is well known as fire as they attack the disease inside the body.

h. ii. Inguva, Ferula foetida, F. narthex, Hingu, Hing, Devil's dung, Asafetida; Hingu-gum is antiseptic, expectorant, anthelmintic, useful in whooping cough; contains (Z)-1-propenyl sec-butyl disulfide (27.7%), (E)-1-propenyl sec-butyl disulfide (20.3%),- means sulfur containing compounds; Asafetida resin is produced by solidifying juice that comes out of cuts made in the plant's living roots. Asafetida is a plant. It has a bad smell and bitter taste. It is commonly used for hysteria, insanity, convulsions, and as a nerve stimulant. Its powder with buttermilk is a very famous Indian home remedy for bloating and to improve digestion power & abdominal and colic pain (Shula).

It is also useful in asthma (Sasarara) and other respiratory disorders. It is useful to restore consciousness (sanjnasthapana). At the same time, it is pungent tasting (Katuskandha) and digestive. Hingu is teekshna (piercing, enters deep tissues) and also cardiac tonic (hrudya). It is a very good natural blood thinning agent. It is also seen to be useful in high blood pressure. Asafetida is pitta-vardhana (increases pitta activity) and good for eyes & improves vision power (Chakshushya). Thus, hingu is used every day in every soups& curries.

h. iii. Hing Patri, Ferula jaescbkeana, Baspika; the roots of this herb are reported to have contraceptive and also anti-implantation activity. Ferujol is a compound in the coumarin family, isolated from this herb. The oil extracted from the leaves possesses mycotoxic property against dermatophytes. Ferujol, isolated from the rhizome, showed abortifacient and anti-implantation activity at a single dose of 0.6 mg/kg in rats. Its galbanum is used in Middle East for rheumatic affections and backache. The roots contain sesquiterpenoids. It is not asafetida, but can cure wounds with its resin and native of Kashmir.

h. iv. Mushini Ginjalu, Srtychnos nux-vomica, Poison Nut, Kuchala, Hemmusti, Mushti Vittulu, Kushti, Musadi, Kupilu; root and fruit contain strychnine and brucine alkaloids; root bark grinded with lime to cure cholera, ulcers; wood used in dysentery, dyspepsia, & fevers; Mushti is used in ayurvedic treatments since the time of Sushruta. Seeds 1-3gms used as medicine or its purified form. Taking nux- vomica for more than a week, or in high amounts of 30 mg or more,-can cause severe side effects like restlessness, dizziness, spasms of jaw and neck, liver failure and death. Dose max for seed powder is below 30 mg.

Preparation: Purification of seeds is a good process. Skin of seeds is removed. It is boiled with milk for 7 days, dried. Then it is fried in ghee and powdered. The roots bark grinded and made pills with lime to cure cholera & ulcers. Its wood powder is used in dysentery, dyspepsia, & fevers. The root and fruit contain most potent alkaloids, strychnine and brucine.

h. v. Musta, Cyperus rotundus, Mustaka, Coco grass, Purplenut sedge, Tungamushti, Nut grass, Tunga musti, Nagarmotha; it is widely used by Ayurveda; it has capacity to penetrate like mustaka every corner and cut the roots of crisis like a rat; it improves lactation, burning sensation, excessive thirst, emmenagogue, anthelmintic, and diaphoretic, Useful in fevers, quench thirst, fevers, solar dermatitis etc., The plant produces rhizomes, tubers, basal bulbs and fibrous roots Musta and Parpataka are the best herbs to relieve fevers. It is absorbent, useful in diarrhea, improves digestion, relieves Ama Dosha, relieves thirst, useful in relieving anorexia; Relieves worm infestation and useful in infected wounds, useful in blood disorders.

h.vi. Yellow nutgrass, Cyperus esculentus: Zulu nut, Ground almond, Tiger nut; Young tubers are white, while older tubers are covered by a yellow outer membrane; Vegetative colonies of its plants are often produced from the tubers and their rhizomes. They are usually preserved by sun drying for about three months before storage. It can be eaten raw, dried, roasted, or grated and can be subjected to further processing. They can be eaten raw, dried, roasted, or grated and can be subjected to further processing. Its uses in cooking and as fuel, baking flour, fish baits; milk is used as a liver tonic, heart stimulant, drank to heal serious stomach pain, to promote normal menstruation, to heal mouth and gum ulcers, used in Ayurvedic medicines and is a powerful aphrodisiac. It is also used in the confectionery industry too.

Note: Cyperus esculentus is called motha and Cyperus rotundus is called Nagarmotha, both are good. Consider Genus Cyperus here.

h. vii. Chitrak, Plumbago zeylanica, Citraka, Chita, Chitra, Leadwort; it- is a useful root in the treatment of – stubborn chronic rheumatoid arthritis, and tumerous growths; root is appetizer, used in skin diseases, piles, made paste with vinegar + milk + salt for leprosy; tincture of bark antipyretic; Citramoolam is a root appetizer, used in skin diseases, piles, made paste with vinegar + milk + salt for leprosy; tincture of bark antipyretic.

viii. Rakta-chitraka, Plumbago indica or P. rosea: Rose colored Leadwort, chiraita, Chita, Lalchita, Erra-chitra-mulamu; The root contains about 0.9% plumbagin. The roots are acrid, vesicant, stimulant, external application for rheumatism & paralytic complaints. The juice of the roots also used as digestive, expectorant, laxative, and treatment of muscular pain. It is also a remedy for secondary syphilitic attack and leprosy conditions. All properties of P. zeylanica stands good for this specie also because, this root is again rich in plumbagin and its derivatives.

6.xii.i. Cardiac tonics, mental coolants & blood pressure lowering: Coolant of brain is a simple herb vishnukranta-discussed in Ganesh puja. In home therapy Allium was discussed.

I. i. Heart pain: It is to be reduced soanf, sunthi and patika-bellam (misri or Gur or sugar) and consume it. Heat sand, tie in cloth and gently keep near heart or lime and honey mixed well and applied. Tella-maddi bark powder @3-5gm boiled and extract given as tea.

I. ii. Cardiac tonics: i. Satapatri, Rosa damascena, Gulab: Damask Rose, Gulab, Persian Rose, Satapatrika, Gulabi; rose petals & sugar consumed as gulkand; rose buds cardiac tonic, remove bile & cold humors. The rose petals are applied externally as astringent and rose flowers are used to make rose water. The water can be stored for five to six months as a diluent in medicine. These flowers contain rose-furan, geraniol and others.

iv. Kat-Gulab, Rosa indica syn Rosa chinensis: Sadagulab; its fruit paste applied to wounds, sprains, injuries, and foul ulcers even. It is cultivated in India. The flowers & to a lesser degree its roots and leaves, are anodyne, emmenagogue, used as uterotonic. The leaves, used in the treatment of arthritis, boils, coughs etc. Rosa chinensis also is a good source of vitamins E and B, antioxidants and the minerals zinc, iron and phosphorous. A tea made from rose hips is an easy and popular way to ingest the health benefits of vitamin C offered by Rosa chinensis. Traditional Indian medicine makes use of the flowers as gulkand, rose water and rose petals for oil. In China flowers are used in treatments for stomach and thyroid problems.

i. ii. Boldo, Plectranthus barbatus, Makandi, Patharchur, Pashan-bhedi, Karmelo; it is synonymous to Coleus forskoli or Indian coleus. Coleus species have been used to treat heart disease, digestive, respiratory, circulatory, nervous disorders, convulsions, spasmodic pain and painful urination. It is a herb used in traditional medicine that may boost testosterone and induce fat loss. It cures infection and also used to treat gastritis and intestinal spasms & nausea.

i. iii. Some more cardio tonics are Digitalis purpurea, Terminalia arjuna, Ephedra geradiana, Stevia rebaudiana, Digitalis plants, Terminalia catappa, Thevetia peruviana, Arnica Montana, Nerium oleander etc. and some are as below.

i.iv. Arjuna: Terminalia arjuna, Arjun Myrobalan, Tellamaddi: cardiotonic, fruit astringent, febrifuge, alterative, externally applied on chronic ulcers, & wounds; locally used as dentifrice, bleeding gums, used in heart diseases and antidote for poison. seed contain astringent substance and tannins (15-30%); its water extract showing promise at improving left ventricle function of the heart without any observable toxicity of side effects when taken at 500mg thrice a day (every 8 hours). The leaf juice can cure earache and the fruit is tonic & deobstruent. The ashes of bark used on scorpion sting. It reduces TB cough also. It cures joint pains, vata, pitta, kapha diseases. Its paste cures injuries also. It contains arjunine, lactones and reducing sugars.

i. v. Vibhitaki, Terminalia belerica, Aksha phala, Beach almond, Karakkai, Bahera, Tandra; In its fruit form, it is used in the popular Indian herbal rasayana treatment triphala. Beleric is a rejuvenative and laxative. It proves beneficial for hair, throat and eyes. Beleric seed oil or fruit paste is applied on swollen parts protects the liver. It is used to respiratory tract infections, cough, and sore throat. It relieves worm infestation also. Its fruit-pericarp is bitter, astringent, tonic, laxative, and antipyretic, used in piles, dropsy and biliousness. Its fruit peri-carp is chewed like a jelly with black pepper and Gur- to clear throat, cough etc., Beleric is a rejuvenative and laxative. Its seeds are narcotic and not used in medicine.

i.vi. Haritaki, Terminalia chebula, Yellow Myrobalan, Harir, Haritaki, Tanikai, Harad; it is a rejuvenator. The flowers are dull white with spikes and can be found at the end of the branches.

The fruit is hard and yellowish green in color, effective in reducing swelling, hastening the healing process and cleansing the wounds and ulcers. Haritaki is having laxative, rejuvenative, purgative and astringent properties. The paste gives relief to the eyelids, in case of conjunctivitis. The bark is cardiotonic and fruit astringent, alterative, externally applied on chronic ulcers & wounds. The fruit decoction also used as gargle & bleeding gums, oral ulcers and sore throat. The bark is diuretic and tonic. The fruit contains tannic acid, chebulinic acid, gallic acid, resin, anthraquinone, sennoside, mucilage and chebulin also.

vii. Badam, Terminalia Catappa, Indian almond, Malabar-almond, Sea-almond; the tree leaves can be used as a diaphoretic, anti-indigestion, and anti-dysentery. Young leaves or scraped bark taken for treating mouth infections, & used to clean fractures. The nuts are edible, taste like almonds and are eaten. The fresh leaves are used in the preparations of medical lotion for leprosy and scabies and the dried leaves are used in the treatment of fish tanks. The leaves, bark and fruits used in dressing of rheumatic joints. The fresh leaves are also used for making steam cooked idly (a south Indian preparation, available all over India now-a-days).

I. viii. Foxglove, Digitalis lanata: Digitalis, Fairy glove, Woolly foxglove, *Grecian-* foxglove, Finger flower; D. purpurea contain less digitoxin content 1.2%, less than D. lanata of Kashmir or that of Australia. So, young Indian plants are better. Some more similar species of Digitalis are Digitalis lanata, Digitalis orientalis & Digitalis nova – all can serve the patients in severe heart conditions. Because of the improved circulation in congestive heart failure caused by fast atrial fibrillation, the kidneys can function better, which stimulates the flow of urine, which lowers the volume of the blood and lessens the load on the heart. But if dose is in excess digitalis is harmful.

Symptoms of digitalis poisoning include nausea, vomiting, severe headache, dilated pupils, problems with eyesight, and convulsions at the worst level of toxicity. As digitalis plant becomes older, the digitoxin concentration goes up.

I. ix. Lady's glove, Digitalis purpurea, Common foxglove, Teelpushpee; A popular ornamental, with purple to pink or white flowers; common foxglove is also a source of digitoxin, used in the heart drug digitalis. Leaves used in certain conditions of heart deteoration. Its extract is a tonic, stimulant and also cures biliousness.

6.xiii.J. Brian activity: One can channelize his thoughts through meditation and concentration.

J1. But, physically in order to achieve high concentration, it needs augmentation by Brahmi (Bacopa monneri) or mandukaparni (Centella asiatica) or Valeriana jatamansi root/fruit powder (tagar or tagada or tegada)- as suggested by an ayurvedic physician.

But increased brain activity means, its increased stimulus through nerves is a must & it needs to be realized through the spinal cord into the body, where Nardostachys jatamansi works. It is available in high altitudes of Himalayas.

J2. Cool your brain or reduce the thought: The other way is to use some drugs of the type – like dhattura (Datura metel/ D. stramonium- also called unmatta, which changed later as ummetta) etc. Or use milder versions like vaca (Acorus calamus), gunja (Abrus precatorius), haridra (Curcuma longa), Ravi (Ficus religiosa) etc. – all act on prolonged use in lower levels. Even asafetida (Ferula narthex) reduces brain activity and cancer risk even.

Another important herb is Ishwari (Arista-lochia indica) that reduces panicky situation and used as dhumrapatra-given during child birth and also called Indian birthwort. Ephedra (Ma Huang) is also a reliable drug with no side effects.

This herb- Ishwari reduces panicky situation and used as dhumrapatra- given during child birth and also called Indian birthwort. Ephedra (Ma Huang) is also a reliable drug with no side effects.

A still lower form is Ummetta or unmatta (literal meaning dozy) or dhattura is Datura innoxia or D. metel. They give Hyoscine etc. alkaloids and its racemic form is atropine (in Genus Atropa and Hyoscyamus). If one is suffering from high blood pressure/tensions, then he naturally need alkaloids from Rauwolfia serpentina, discussed later. If spinal-cord is problematic, then take jatamansi, (Nardostachys jatamansi DC, Nardostachys grandiflora). Another set is of Genus Valeriana, that are brain coolants through spinal cord.

But, the immediate or on the spot cooling-way is to suppress by the use some drugs of the type surapana (alcohol), opium, bhang or lysergic acid derivatives etc. Now many psychotropic drugs are available, but they also use morphine injections for immediate relief (after surgery). Details are as below.

J2.i. Patala agandi, Rauwolfia serpentina, Java devil pepper, Serpentine Roots, Snake root, Insanity herb, Chandrika, Sarpagandha, Patalagaruda, Chandra: it increases uterine movements; root hypnotic, reduces blood pressure, remedy for bowel affections; it has yohimbine alkaloids.

It contains serpentine alkaloids (reserpine and others) that reduce blood pressure, depresses activity of central nervous system and act as hypnotic. The juice of leaves used for removal of opacious cornea of eyes. It increases uterine transactions. Specie is also available and most common in AP.

J2.ii. Bhutjati, Nardostachys jatamansi DC, Nardostachys grandiflora, Jatamansi, Bhoothajata, Thapaswini, Muskroot, Balchar, Spikenard, Muskroot, Balchar, Sambul lateeb; Bhutjati means- an uncombed devil hair. it is a flowering plant of the Valerian family that grows in the Himalayas. Root aromatic, bitter, tonic, stimulant, antiseptic, hysteria, palpitation of heart, used in epilepsy treatment. The spinal cord which sends mind's signals to the body through it. Jatamansi is hence, a natural brain nervine tonic and a memory enhancer, which has calming, peacefulness and relaxation in its features. It is available in the form of root, oil and powder. It is prescribed against stress, spasm, epilepsy, convulsion and hysteria. It ensures good cardiac condition. It helps to provide vitality, vigor and strength to the body through a good for the nervous system.

J2.iii. Belladonna, Atropa acuminata or Atropa belladonna: Deadly nightshade Baccifère, Belladonna, Bella done, Angurhafa, Sag-angur; Belladonna means beautiful eyes in Greek and used in homeopathy; used in homeopathy; anodyne, sedative, antispasmodic, and for irritable bowels.

It is poisonous, contains atropine 0.08% to 0,15% in leaves, & 0.3 to 0.8% in roots. The drug obtained by this plant through their young leaves and flowers. It acts as strong drug which used to relieve acute abdominal pain. It is narcotic, sedative, anodyne and poisonous. Atropine is a racemic form of tropane alkaloids.

J2.iv. Henbane, Hyoscyamus Niger, Black henbane, Stinking nightshade, Khurasani ajwain, Parseek yawani; leaves sedative, anodyne, antispasmodic, employed in irritable conditions and spasmodic affections, seeds toxic, astringent to bowels; contains hyoscyamine and hyoscine; leaves sedative, anodyne, antispasmodic, employed in irritable conditions and spasmodic affections, seeds toxic, astringent to bowels. Its leaves and leaf oil are used as sedative, narcotic and anodyne. It cures intestinal spasms too.

J2.v. Dhattura (Datura innoxia or Datura metel); the natural Indian alternative is containing L-isomer of alkaloids and is readily available on roadside bushes. It already discussed in Ganesh puja.

J2.vi. Brahma-Manduki, Centella asiatica, Hydro cotyle asiatica, Brahma-Buti, Gotukola, Mandukaparni, Coin wort, Penny weed, Spade leaf, Bar manimuni, Asiatic Pennywort, Pegaga; its leaves tonic, and cures diseases of skin both internally and externally; GotuKola is a rejuvenator and nervine recommended for nervous disorders, including epilepsy and senility.

Its extract is a nervine tonic, used in leprosy, asthma, given to cure brain diseases. It is of bitter taste and also a tonic. It is a blood and nerve cleaner and contains asiaticoside, centellin, asiaticin, and centellicin etc.

J2. Vii. Brahmi is another wild growing herb for improving mental ability.

J2. Viii. Black Cohosh, Cimicifuga racemosa, Actaea racemosa, Sheng Ma, Black Snakeroot, Bugbane, Squawroot, kattu-k-kolinci, Baringtonia racemosa- the rhizome is mild purgative, insect resistant; Recognized for its mild sedative and anti-inflammatory activity, black cohosh can help with hot flashes and thus emmenagogue, a trusted drug in America. It cures anxiety, purgative and also insect resistant. It is also useful to treat joint pain, pain, and pain in pregnancy and labor.

Black cohosh has also been used to treat influenza, smallpox, acute rheumatism, headache, cough, and other nervous system disorders; it contains cimicifugic acid, & several polyphenols like protocatechuic acid, protocatechualdehyde, p-coumaric acid, methyl caffeate, ferulic acid, ferulate-1-methyl ester, isoferulic acid etc.

J2.ix. Sugandha bala, Valeriana wallichi, Valeriana jatamansi, Grandhi Tagaramu, Indian valerian, Tagger, Mushk bala, Tagara, All-heal, Amantilla, Baldrian, Great Wild, Risha-wala, Valerian Phu, Tagar; It is a perennial flowering plant, with heads of sweetly scented pink or white flowers that bloom in the summer. Indian valerian is used as anodyne, antispasmodic, aromatic, calmative, carminative, diuretic, expectorant, nervine, relaxant, sedative, stimulant and tranquilizer; root yield 0.5 to 2% volatile oil; root also contain large amounts water solubles;

The rhizomes are greenish-brown in color and hard and tough internally. Valerian flower extracts were used as a perfume even in the 16th century. Medicine is made from the root. In manufacturing, the extracts and oil made from valerian are used as flavoring in foods and beverages.

J2.x. Tagar, Valeriana officinalis, Great wild valerian, Garden Heliotrope, All-heal, Anantilla, Velandswurt, Valerian; Valerian is also used for conditions connected to anxiety and psychological stress including nervous asthma, hysterical states, excitability, fear of illness (hypochondria), headaches, migraine, and stomach upset.

Its medicine is made from the root, most commonly used for sleep disorders, especially the inability to sleep (insomnia). It is frequently combined with hops (that used in beer brew), lemon balm, or other herbs that also cause drowsiness. In manufacturing, the extracts and oil made from valerian are used as flavoring in foods and beverages.

J2. xi. Another mental coolant is morphine alkaloids supplied as opium or nalla mandu, isolated from Papaver somniferum or khas-khas (discussed in spices), used in post operative treatments.

J2. xii. The next is Hashish or Charas or bhang, hemp, Cannabis sativa which contains psychoactive cannabinoids and it is used since Krita yuga where Shiva is offered bhang as a mental coolant. It is used extensively as medication since ages, but records exist from 8th century. Herb is antipyretic & analgesic, and also anti-inflammatory. The herb Cannabis contains more than 400 compounds.

Its compound Cannabidiol has Anxiolytic, Antipsychotic, Analgesic, Anti-inflammatory, Antioxidant, Antispasmodic, Anti-emetic, Antifungal, Anticonvulsant, and Antidepressant too.

6.XIV.K. Fever curatives: rojmari, ulatkhambal, camel thorn, kalmegh, turmeric, daruharidra, Cinchona bark etc.,-are powerful and specific fever curative herbs. What are the types of fevers & how their treatments are differing?

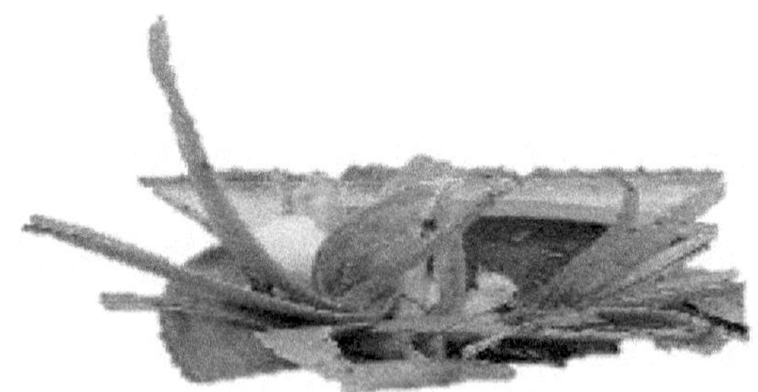

(kalabanda)

6.c. Some more complicated treatments: Fevers: Exhaustion or exertion, overwork also leads to fever- that gets cured by rest. In my subject preview, I had mentioned cow dung treatment. So, serve a cow if you are healthy and if you are a TB patient, serve a goat- ayurvedic recommendation.

It usually eliminates root problems that lead to fevers. Thus, coming to some of these fevers' treatments were suggested in a simple way then.

Note: At present, the people have ignored the use of green leafy vegetables- which if consumed daily no problems in the digestive tract.

India is blessed with lot of variety of leafy vegetables. At least consume leafy vegetables-once/twice a week — as it can produce cleaning effect in GI Tract as discussed earlier.

During my childhood days, my fever was treated with apc tablets (adenine-pethidine-caffeine) and later came- sulphadiazine.

Type of Fevers: But there are fevers which vary, viz., high temperature fevers, fever due to indigestion, fever with cold, pneumonia, malaria, chicken pox etc. But every fever is associated with indigestion or indisposed liver- a vital point to remember. If liver is treated, many fevers vanish.

In Saka way of counting the years, I have observed an interesting phenomenon- after 60 years, some epidemic is to strike. Thus, in the year sarvari (sara-means an arrow; ari means enemy- means epidemic is to come) and covid-19 struck!

Previously, cholera, plague, chicken pox or small pox were struck after some @ 50-year intervals. Then the people were isolated to die- with lack of medicine. Thus, even astrology indicates the upcoming epidemic.

In the olden days these fevers are defined in a different way. I took some details of family predecessor's views, and also his father's note became handy. Fever including typhoid fever were handled with herbs.

My maternal-grandfather during his childhood suffered it and consumed a dozen ripe bananas which cleared his entire digestive tract of residual bacilli and became normal followed by spice rich food supplements.

But this may not suit to all persons. Typhoid fever needs clearance of accumulated food that harp bacilli. Present typhoid has several variants-making modern physician – a must. So, one uses modern antibiotics now.

k. i. old methods are raavi or ravi leaf plus maredu leaf and tulasi leaf if consumed @5gms thrice daily for @ one week- to eliminate root of fever and spice rich rasam cures the rest!

Unusual fevers: These fevers were classified (@30) for treatment by our family predecessor, but no longer used now. Below, I give some follow-up treatments.

k.ii. For Intermittent Fevers

- Bhumya-malaki/nela- vemu; black pepper or maricha (miriyalu); Neem leaf steaks after removal of leaves; Burada-gondi (or pigweed or Boerhaavia diffusa); Guduci (or somida or tippa-teega) and processed as below procedure.

Taken all herbs in equal amounts powdered and mixed. Take 20gm mixture added 20x32 ml= 640 ml and allowed to reduce to half a volume, liquid squeezed through muslin cloth and given at a single dose of 14 ml for three days.

k.iii. For vata fevers: Guduchi, nela vemu, dried ginger, tunga gaddalu (roots that came out of the soil)- all mixed powders 2gm each taken with honey or as extract as previous procedure.

k.iv. For sleshma fevers: Gandha- kachuram, sunthi, pippallu, maricha, vasaka, gantu-baranki-chettu (it is Clerodendrum serratum)-used.

k.v. For poisonous fevers: Vishnu madhu-kuttu (probably mul-hathi), katuki, karakkai, chedu-potla (patola), tunga mushti (tunga-gaddalu)- all powdered and mixed and used.

k. vi. For sannipata fevers: nela-vemu, maricha, katuki, vepa vennelu, tippa teega, duradagondi (dulagondi or Mucuna pruriens) roots, all powders well mixed and stored. For all these five preparations, the powders can be given with a maximum dose of one tola per day, but for sannipata fevers, more has to be given as suggested by the physician. Probably sannipata is improperly prepared metal- poisoning.

k.vii. For thirst during fevers: Parpataka, vetiver, duradagondi (Kapi kachhu), Chandan,- all mixed-2gm.x3/day.

k.viii. For thirst during fevers: Rudraksh, Vishnu madhukam, pogadam, arka stem (with pericarp removed), Sindhava salt, lime juice, all mixed powders about half gram, thrice or five times/day till cure.

k.ix. Fever with vata: Arka roots and sunthi- both separately powdered and reduced to a fine paste with water or milk and allow it to dry on skin, along the spinal cord or on to the chest. Apply twice a day.

k.x. If there is cough during the fevers, karakkai flowers about one eighth of tola (1.5 Gms), cloves one tola, maricha one tola,- all made to Kashaya and distributed to four doses.

Now, let us look into some fever curative herbs

k.xi. Gandana or Rojmari or Achillea millefolium plays a vital role, in curing fevers or injuries but sparingly available in India and widely available in Europe up to Canada. (Discussed in Ganapati puja).

k.xii. Ulat khamb (meaning- remove the rug), Abroma augusta: Pisacha karpasa, Gogu, Konda gogu, Devil's Cotton are different names for this plant. Abroma Augusta extract recovers from fever relieves headache. The root bark is used as emetic, uterotonic, used in dysmenorrhea also. It contains alkaloids- abromine and others in 0.01%. Not advised during pregnancy.

Medical advice is necessary for its use in children and during lactation. Root and bark contain gum, fixed oil, resin, choline, friedelin, abroma-sterol, betaine, beta-sitosterol, stigmasterol, digitonide, polysaccharide and magnesium salts. It also contains sugars like, rhamnose, arabinose, mannose, galactose, and glucose – and also many others.

The leaves contain taraxasterol and its acetates also. It is used for gynecological disorders, infertility treatment and amenorrhea.

k.xiii. Quinine bark, Cinchona officinalis, Peruvian bark, Kunina (quina), Cinchona, Curappattai, Jvarapatta, Kina kina, China bark; C. ledgeriana, C. Robusta and C. succiruba; All Cinchona species above contain quinine; cinchona cures mild attacks of cold, swine flu, fever and even used for the treatment of malaria. It is rich in alkaloids including quinidine, quinine, cinchonine and cinchonidine; The bark is stripped from the tree, dried, and powdered for medicinal uses. Cinchona is used for increasing appetite, promoting the release of digestive juices, and treating stomach troubles. It is also used for regulating varicose veins and cleaning blood vessels. Some people use to treat cancer of mouth and throat diseases, spleen and muscle cramps. Cinchona is used even in eye lotions, and is an astringent. Cinchona extract is also applied to grow hair and cure hemorrhoids.

k.xiv. Neelini, Indigofera tinctorea, Indigo, Neel, Neelamari, Black Henna, True Indigo, Nilika, Nili, Aviri, Nilam, Neela, Neeli-mandu; leaf juice prophylactic, & used in hydrophobia, ext. of plant given in epilepsy; root used in hepatitis & scorpion sting; hexane extract of plant showed

21 chemical compounds, alpha-linolenic acid being 47.03%, indigoferin etc. Indigo was a popular dye during the Middle Ages. It has been used medicinally as an emetic; the Chinese used the plant to purify the liver, reduce inflammation and fever and to alleviate pain. The blue dye is produced during the fermentation of the leaves, which is commonly accomplished with caustic soda or sodium hydrosulfite. Indigo also has been used as a nematicide and treatment for a range of ills including ovarian or stomach cancer.

k.xv. Stinging nettle, Urtica dioica radix: Common nettle, stinging nettle, Bichu, Kandadli, chorat, Nettle leaf; flowering plant, contains lecithin; It is a perennial plant for rheumatic complaints. It is a century old medicine for treating allergies, fever and inflammation. Herb is used in decongestants, anti-histamines, allergy shots.

- Bichu, Urtica parviflora, Bichubooti, Common nettle, Shisoon, stinging nettle; Although the fresh leaves have stinging hairs, thoroughly drying or cooking them destroys these hairs. Hence, only young leaves should be used because older leaves develop gritty particles called cystoliths which act as an irritant to the kidneys. A very nutritious food, high in vitamins and minerals, it makes an excellent spinach substitute and can also be added to soups and stews. Nettle beer is brewed from the young shoots.

k.xiv. Rhubarb, Rheum emodi; Himalayan-rhubarb, Amlavetasa, Revantchini; is used as tonic, diuretic and to treats fever, cough & indigestion, strong laxative; The root and stem of the plant are rich in anthraquinones, such as emodin and Rhein. Rhubarb is used as purgative and astringent tonic. Its stimulating effect is visible in combination with aspirin. Rhubarb is also useful in curing atonic dyspepsia. These substances are cathartic and laxative, which is also the reason why rhubarb acts a slimming agent.

Rhubarb is used for making jams and sauce. It is also cooked with strawberries or apples as a sweetener or with stem or root ginger, to make various types of jams and sausages. The leaves of the plant are used to make an effective organic insecticide for leaf-eating insects, such as cabbage caterpillars, aphids, peach and cherry slug etc., and amlavetasa leaves are used for treating fatal poisoning. The herb contains tannins, emodin and hydroxy- anthracene derivatives, & chrysophanol glycosides.

k.xvii. Reebanda ciinii, Naattu raevalchini, Rheum australe; Himalayan rhubarb, Red-veined pie plant; Rheum is a genus of about 60 perennial plants in the family. Many Rheum species have food and medicinal uses, besides having ornamental qualities and this includes R. acuminatum, R. Alexandrea, R. australe and R. kialense. Himalayan rhubarb is a perennial plant and native to central Asia. Rhubarb is used as purgative and astringent tonic. Its stimulating effect, combined with aspirin properties, renders it especially useful in atonic dyspepsia.

k.xviii. Chiraita, Swertia chirata, Nilavemu, Kairata, Nilavembu, Nelaveppa; wp-bitter, tonic, febrifuge, laxative, contain chiratin, ophaelic acid- derivatives of salicylic acid- thus anodyne too, contains xanthone and flavanol glycosides. The Ayurvedic medicine Swertia Chirata is called a tridosha balancing. All parts of the plants can be used for making either a dried herb or powder. It's bitter, hot, pungent, and dry thus making it good for most conditions.

The herb, Chirata is used in treating fever, constipation, and loss of appetite, intestinal worms, skin diseases, and even cancer. Swertia is a powerful anti-inflammatory and used for rheumatoid arthritis. Swertia has the ability to lower blood sugar, by stimulating insulin production in pancreatic cells.

k.xix. Banafsha, Viola odorata Flores: Banaksa, Banafsha, Wood violet, Nilapuspa, Garden violet, Vanapsa, Sweet violet, Banapsa; best medicine for fevers, plant antipyretic, diaphoretic, febrifuge; flowers emollient, used in biliousness & lung troubles; root emetic; contain methyl salicylate and rutin; even leaf tops have salicylates; Its flowers and leaves are edible.

It is used in treating cough, asthma, fever with burning sensation, body-ache etc. Young leaves and flower buds- raw or cooked. They make a very good salad, their mild flavor enabling them to be used in bulk whilst other stronger-tasting leaves can then be added to give more flavors.

A tea can be made from the leaves. It is used as an ingredient in many herbal cough syrups; best herbal medicine for fevers, plant antipyretic, diaphoretic and febrifuge. The flowers are emollient and used in biliousness & lung troubles. Its roots are emetic. It contains methyl salicylates and rutin. Even its leaf tops have salicylates.

k.xx. White Violet, Viola pilosa, Viola pogonantha, Banafshah, Ghatte, Smooth-Leaf pansy; Smooth-Leaf White Violet is found in the Himalayas, is a perennial herb. More than 40% material readily dissolves in 90% alcohol, many not tested-but used as extract. It is also called banafshah. More herbs like nelavemu, nela-usiri, wintergreen, Ficus species, bach, mango, etc. were reputed fever curatives then.

k.xxi. Stress: Even distress signals exist with injury or stress or some poison in the form of acetyl choline, adrenaline, epi-nephrine, nor-epi-nephrine, or arachidonic acid etc. These molecules are gradually destroyed by bilwa, mango, fever curative herbs or methyl salicylate rich herbs or spice rich rasam etc. used then. But sometimes in a chronic patient, it takes months to reduce these toxins. It is here metal complexes are useful.

6.xv.l. Diabetes cure: Diabetes in Greek language means a fountain of sugar. Diabetes – or prameha in ayurveda did not find importance in the list of diseases in the Glossary on medicinal plants by CSIR (Chopra and Chopra), i.e., at the time of pre independence era. But later it blew out of proportions and after independence with increased money circulation the disease-diabetes had blown out of proportions.

According to Dr. Bajaj (in his interview with Vivek Sharma on DD-1 on 8th July 1998) – there will be 60 million cases of diabetes by the year 2000 and it will go up further. This is because; modern technology had increased sedentary habits. A fat body is an open gate for diabetes – is the pet quotation.

How? According to my understanding, the body begins its way of expression by consuming food and releasing products like NADPH, NADH, ATP etc., What happens to an alcoholic or a smoker or an opium consumer or a hallucinated drug patient, the levels of cyclic AMP can be or should be high – as it is habit forming. There could be an excess release of this molecule means the patient has some addictions and the protein actions in that patient become sluggish.

When the body unit cell is looked into, it- as a breakup has A, B, C, & D cells. If glucose levels are high, D- cells release somatostatin, which signals B-cell to release insulin and C-cells release C-peptide. In fact, in good old days, C-peptide is estimated to be a quantitative measure of insulin. If the body glucose levels are low, A cells send a signal as glucagon from it sends message to block the release of insulin on one side and glycogen formation on the other side.

L. i. Diabetes in ayurveda: In India prameha is the name of the group wherein diabetes (madhumeh) is one part of that group.

In 1980, there appeared a good article by Dr. H. M. Chandola and S.N. Tripathi (J.Ay.Sid.1980, 224-238) who clarified that in ayurveda there are ten sub-types of kaphaja prameha, six sub-types of paittika prameha and four sub-types of vattika prameha, but when viewed in summation, they are udakameha (Diabetes insipidus), Sandrameha (Chyluria), sukrameha (spermatorrhea), sikatameha (lithuria) kalameha or raktameha or manjishta meha— combinedly called hematuria, haridra meha (biliuria), vasa meha (lipuria), majja meha (gonorrhea), Ikshu meha (glucosuria), sheet meha renal-glucosuria) and finally Madhu meha (diabetes).

In fact, all these prameha give the levels of diabetic damage in the patient and each level is separately treated in ayurveda, where prevention is much better than cure.

L. ii. Sugar reduction: The newspaper, Indian Express carried diabetes awareness carried two series of articles. One set- series by

A. Ramachandran starting from 21ˢᵗ August, 1993-for about six weeks on diabetes and later another set-on living with diabetes by Dr. M.P. Agarwal starting from 16ᵗʰ Jan, 1994 for about 6 weeks. Summations of some vital points are as below.

i.   By daily walk of about four kilometers, plus reduction of fat in diet, avoiding high calorie diet (sweets, sugar, potatoes & rice), but with enough yoghurt and increased salad diet.

ii. Do exercises or walk four kms a day and accept sugar free instead sugar. Here, the Keir's triangle determines the extent of sweetness in a molecule or in a sugar substitute as suggested by modern literature. But how far they are safe- is a big question.

L.ii. According to Ramachandran- syndrome X is most common in Indians and even more prevalent in NRI Indians.

L.iii. According to Dr. Agarwal, a strict adherence to diet restrictions can manage a diabetic better.

L.iv. In my opinion, diabetes spurt as people stopped hard works like hand weaving of clothes, walking long distances, use electric grinders instead age-old stone grinding for pulverizing grains, even wood cutting- thanks to the mechanization.

Hence, consume less food. Here hunger is proportional to the salt consumed. It is said that there are three enemies to the body, namely sweet, oil fried stuff and excess salt in food consumption. If one reduces them and add fruit and salads to diet, there is less acid formation and less or genuine hunger.

L.v. Since olden days, the vegetable kakara (Momordica charantia) serves as food supplement cum treatment. In Odisha Sun dried vegetable chips are supplied as salad during lunch on the roadside restaurants even today, which is missing in the modern inns.

L.vi. The Ayurvedic practice is podapatri (Gymnema Silvestre), wherein the leaves are chewed repeatedly till the jaw refuses to move. It means the sugar level is low & tastes like sand in the mouth.

L.vii. Or use kalmegh or nelavemu with punarnava (Boerhaavia diffusa) is deeply beneficial as pancreas may get activated in natural diets.

L.viii. Gandhian diet, if added to it in the form of neem leaves into the food, the benefits are far reaching.

L. ix. Diabetic coma: In India the bark of raktachandan (Pterocarpus marsupium) is suggested emergency measure.

In the good old days two dolls of raktachandan were used to be gifted as above to the newly married couple. They prevent diabetic coma. They say these dolls rescue life in emergencies at least five times where the doll is soaked in water & the fluid is given to the patient.

The real problem is that now these Idols may not be of raktachandan (probably of kamala tree), hence not anti-diabetic. Now-a-days diabetic wooden cups are made available on net and can be used @five occasions with hot water to rescue from diabetic coma. Treatment of diabetes: There are more plants and vegetables available in India to tackle diabetes on a long run.

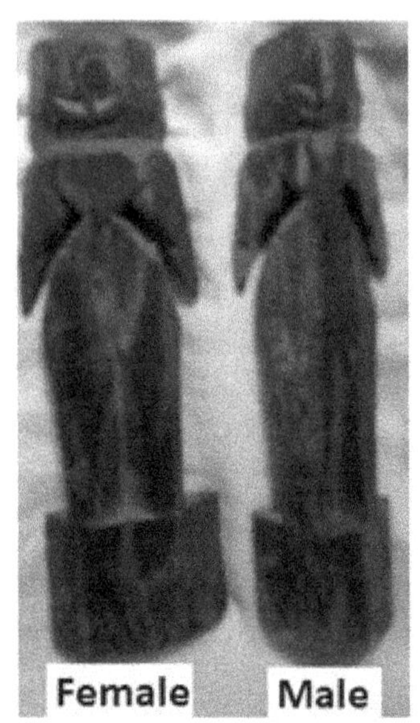

These are small dolls used to be given as a gift in good old days. They serve as an emergency measure to make person recover from diabetic coma.

So, minimization of diabetic effects is more practical, as mentioned earlier and some can be as below.

Prameha can be treated with svarasa of leaf of bilva (bael), svarasa of guduchi-10ml, thrice/day; or powder of- gurmar, (Gymnema Silvestre) leaves 2gm. or powder of satavari 25g. + 250ml cow milk, twice a day; or powdered seed of jambu1-2g. Thrice a day; Now-a-days many ayurveda companies offer goli or tablets or juice bottles for cure.

The treatment of diabetes is established in the modern medicine into two types, Insulin Dependent Diabetes mellitus (IDDM) and Non-insulin- DDM. In case of IDDM, cannot be handled through food, but with insulin shots. With chemical work involving production of tolbutamide type sulphonyl ureas or glibenclamide type structures as sugar reducers, NIDDM is brought to control. Plus, there is large number of sugar substitutes also- thanks to the modern developments.

L. x. Herbs-anti-diabetic: In India, the following herbs were suggested to be useful in NIDDM patients. They are Abutilon indicum, Acacia catechu, Ageratum conyzoides, Allium sativum (garlic), Alpinia galangal, Andrographis paniculata, Azadirachta indica, Gymnema Silvestre (poda Patri), Mangifera indica (mango), Momordica charantia (kakara), Myristica fragrans, Murraya koenigii (curry leaves), Pterocarpus marsupium, Syzygium cumini (neredu), Terminalia belerica (karakkai), Terminalia chebula (tanikai), Tinospora cordifolia (somida or giloe), Trigonella foenum-graecum (methi), etc.,

In India, the following herbs were also considered to be useful in NIDDM patients. They are Abutilon indicum, Acacia catechu, Ageratum conyzoides, Allium sativum (garlic), Alpinia galangal, Andrographis paniculata, Azadirachta indica, Gymnema sylvestre (poda patri), Mangifera indica (mango), Momordica charantia (kakara), Myristica fragrans, Murraya koenigii (curry leaves), Pterocarpus marsupium, Syzygium cumini (neredu), Terminalia belerica (karakkai), Terminalia chebula (tanikai), Tinospora cordifolia (somida or giloe), Trigonella foenum-graecum (methi), etc.,

"Here most of them are also liver stimulating herbs. This means even liver tonics can check some problems of diabetes in initial levels and even can help in the regeneration of pancreas".

A. Fenugreek, Trigonella foenum-graecum, Methre, menthi-kura; It is cultivated in India as a semiarid crop. Its seeds and leaves are common ingredients in dishes and have been used as a culinary ingredient since ancient times. Trigonella is antidiabetic with metformin in its seeds in good amounts, discussed as a spice.

B. Jangli-kuth, Arctium lappa radix, Arctium, Burdock, Arctium minus, Arctium tomentosum; is diuretic, diaphoretic, roots contain 45% inulin- useful for diabetics, taken by mouth to treat colds, cancer, anorexia, stomach and intestinal complaints, joint pain, gout, bladder infections, diabetes; Burdock roots contain mucilage, sulfurous acetylene compounds, polyacetylenes and bitter guaianolides;- all are commonly called as burdock; the root is sometimes used as food. The root, leaf, and seed are used to make medicine. People take burdock to increase urine flow, kill germs and reduce fever.

It is used to treat nervosa, gastrointestinal complaints, rheumatism, acne, gout, bladder infections complications of syphilis, eczema and even psoriasis. Burdock lowers blood pressure and liver diseases. Some people use burdock as aphrodisiac. The high biofilm inhibition efficiency of burdock leaf fraction was probably due to the combination action of phenolic compounds present in the fraction. It contains p-coumaric acid, cynarine, quercetin and also luteolin.

L.xi. Kasni, Cichorium intybus, Chicory, Kasini, Hinduba, Kasani; it is a perennial plant with salad leaf; used in fevers, wounds of diabetes; used in enlargement of spleen; root stomachic, appetizer; contains lactucin, & chicorin; it is a coffee substitute, vegetable crop and tonic, used in fevers, root stomachic & emmenagogue; the root contained @ 40% inulin, thus is suitable for diabetics. It is a liver tonic and also for cough cure.

L.xii. Gurmar, Gymnema sylvestre, Chakkarakolli, Ram's horn, Dhuleti, Mardashingi, Podapatri, Australian cow-plant, Madhu-nashini; leaves chewed in glycaemia to bring down sugar levels; it is also used in treating eye diseases, allergies, constipation, cough dental caries, obesity, stomach ailments, and viral infections.

Gymnema is used in emetic, expectorant, contains gymnemic acid and anthraquinone derivatives; the constituents isolated from its leaves include gymnemasin- A, B, C, and D and alkaloids. It also contains a number of saponins like gymnemic acid, deacyl-gymnemic acid, gymnemagenin, 23-hydroxyl- nogispinogenin, and gymnestrogenin, besides-betaine, choline, and trimethylamine.

L.xiii. Raktachandan, Pterocarpus marsupium, Malabar kino, Indian kino tree, Vijaya Sar, Vengisa- is popular in diabetes and obesity which contains 75% kino-tannic acid; Gum, leaf juice cure earache; reduce the sugar level or cools blood (rakta-chandanam) and makes him recover from diabetic coma.

The most common uses of Pterocarpus in modern herbal medicine include helping support the body's natural ability to manage and regulate blood sugar levels. It is also used for bleeding and toothaches and useful for skin affections. It is a gigantic tree.

- Diabetes (part of prameha): it can be treated with svarasa of leaf of bilva (bael), svarasa of guduchi-10ml, thrice/day; or powder of madhunasani-(gurmar, Gymnema sylvestre) leaves 2gm. or powder of satavari 25g. + 250 ml cow milk, twice a day; or powdered seed of jambu1-2g. Thrice a day; Now-a-days many ayurveda companies offer goli or tablets or juice bottles for cure. Authors from Jamnagar university had reviewed on sugar reducing herbs long back.

6.xvi.m. Tonic Herbs

m. i. Jeoputra, Putranjiva roxburghii, Putranjivaka, Jeoputra means live till have a grandson or long live. Its wp is a tonic, used for the treatment of eye disorders, burning sensation, elephantiasis, and habitual abortions. As a medicated feed, it is uterine tonic. Bark used as medicine; *its* fruit & leaves also are used in rheumatism.

m. ii. Moduga, Butea monosperma, Palas, Plaksha, Forest flare; Palash tree is also known as 'flame of the forest' because of its red-colored flowers. The gum obtained from the tree is rich in gallic acid and tannic acid and is referred to as Bengal kino gum. The leaves of the Butea monosperma are used as ingredients of tonics and aphrodisiacs and are also helpful in arresting bleeding or secretion.

Used to cure diabetes, eye related diseases. It appears to mostly be recommended as a general health tonic and for the treatment of liver disorders. The seeds are anthelmintic, leaves & flowers astringent. The flowers aphrodisiac and the bark & seed used in snakebite. Contains butene etc.

m. iii. Ippa, Madhuca indica, Butter tree, Mahua, Mohwa, Irippa, Madhuka, Ippe, Yappa; madhuca means sweet bearing (flowers)- traditionally worshipped as Srimukhalinga- used as cooling agent, tonic, aphrodisiac, and astringent, demulcent; The barks, flowers, leaves as well as the seeds of the plant are used in medicinal drugs. The flowers are edible and sweet in taste.

The flowers yield distilled spirit which is astringent, tonic, nutritive & appetizing. Hence, they serve it as herbal tonic. It is used in cough and also regarded as cooling. The dried flowers used as fomentation in orchitis for sedative effect.

The dried flowers are fried in ghee and eaten by persons suffering from piles. The bark is used in decoction as astringent, tonic and fish poison. The leaves of mahua are effective in the treatment of eczema. The extracted oil of madhuca is reported to be emollient, used in rheumatism and headache.

m. iv. Ginseng, Panax ginseng: root tonic, fever curative, adaptogen,- is one of the most well – known herbs in traditional Chinese medicine. The root is believed to be good for your lungs, strengthen your spleen and stomach, benefit your heart and calm your mind. Panax ginseng might decrease higher levels of blood sugar.

In diabetics medications are used to lower blood sugar. It is a cardiac stimulant and aphrodisiac. It is also used for common cold and flu, heart failure, high blood pressure, quality of life, wrinkled skin, and to slow the aging process. This might cause side effects such as anxiousness, headache, restlessness, and insomnia.

m.v. Pseudo-ginseng, Aralia cachemerica: Aralia caesia, Aralia californica, Aralia racemosa and Aralia nudicaulis- all have similar properties.; Pseudo- ginseng is an excellent tonic and a good substitute for Panax- ginseng – as a tonic, aphrodisiac, stimulant, used in dyspepsia, vomiting, expectorant and antipyretic; Aqueous Alcoholic extract of root shows anti-hyperglycemic activity. The plant Aralia cachemerica is reported to contain Octadec-6-enoic acid, 8- primara-14, 15-diene-19-oic acid, Aralosides A&B nonane, a hexacosane derivative, petroselinic acid, stigmasterol and sitosterol.

Very recently two disaccharides, Glucopyranosyl – O (1,2) fructo-furanoside (sucrose) {1} and Gluco-pyranosyl-O-(1,4) gluco-pyranoside (Maltose) {2} have been isolated from its roots. Plant also possesses antibacterial properties. Aralia nudicaulis is distributed in North America, mainly in Canada, shows anti-cancer activity.

m.vi. Ashwagandha, Withania somnifera, Sleepy-nightshade, Indian ginseng and Poison gooseberry, winter cherry: The plant has been used as an aphrodisiac, liver tonic, anti-inflammatory agent, and more recently to treat asthma, ulcers, insomnia, it is a tonic and aphrodisiac and used in anxiety, cognitive and neurological disorders, inflammation, and Parkinson's disease.

m. vii. Even pomegranate fruit is a good as a tonic.

6.xvii.n. If skin affections: Burns, allergies and sores: The cure is with Garlic., Urtica dioica (again Sulphur rich); Rosemary (Rosemary essential oil is a home remedy & used as antioxidant, and anti-inflammation); rojmari for burns; Turmeric (haldi), Moor-konda- leaves and flowers used for bedsores and wounds treatment; Bryophyllum pinnatum used for boils, swelling, insect-bite, burns and wounds; Datura metel, Datura stramonium, Hyoscyamus Niger etc., Leukoderma develops, the cure is with Aristolochia indica, Ammi majus, Heracleum candicans etc., Leukoderma cure: Aristolochia indica, Ammi majus, Heracleum candicans etc.,

n2. Corns/warts if develop

n. i. Papaya: Carica papaya; Boppai, its fruit — raw used as a vegetable and fruit consumed. But fruit is abortifacient. The leaf juice used for warts, corns, tumors, and thickened skin; the roots used for treating uterine cancers; contains collagen can destroy cells.

n. ii. Aswatha, Ficus religiosa, Ravi, Pipal, Bodhi, Pippala, Peepul, Buddha; peepal or pippala is astringent, used in gonorrhea. Its fruit is laxative, seeds cooling, and alterative. Its leaves and young shoots are purgative. The infusion of the bark is internally given to cure scabies and rashes on the skin. Its leaves and delicate shoots are used for skin diseases. Also improves digestion. Some more Ficus species are as below.

n. iii. Banyan, Ficus benghalensis, Nyagrodha, Vata, Marri; infusion of bark used in diabetes, seeds coolant, tonic, soft shoot or bark tonic, antiseptic, astringent, diaphoretic, The sap of banyan cure cracks on the skin and also applied on abscesses, The latex with milk cures rheumatism, piles and also lumbago. Marri bark infusion used in diabetes, dysentery, nervous disorders, burning sensation, known for anti- hyperglycemic or antidiabetic, seeds coolant, tonic, buds, leaves, fruits and latex are used in seminal weakness; contains phytosterols, anthocyanidin derivatives.

n. iv. Udumbara, Ficus glomerata, Medi, Atti- has several therapeutic uses in the traditional system. All parts of the plant are involved in medicinal cure.

n. v. Cluster fig, Ficus racemosa Linn; is another popular medicinal plant in India,-has long been used in Ayurveda and used as above. But unlike the banyan, it has no aerial roots; It is called goolar, atti, & medi.

n.vi. Edible fig, Ficus carica, Anjir, Anjeer, Common Fig; the latex of fig has been used in traditional herbal medicine to treat skin viral infections and even warts.

n. vii. Brahma's Banyan, Rough banyan, Sandpaper fig, Ficus exasperata, Ficus asperrima, Karasana; the tree is widely used as a source of sandpaper. The extracts from the tree used to treat as anti-ulcer.

viii. Bomma-medi, Ficus hispida Linn, kathumar, Gobla, kakodumbara, Hairy fig, Devil fig; used in the treatment of ulcers, diabetes, dysentery, psoriasis, anemia, piles and jaundice.

n. ix. Kallaravi, Ficus arnottiana, Indian Rock Fig, Waved-leaved fig tree, Wild pipal; Used in wound healing and its bark used in skin diseases;

n. x. Darbha, Kusha – Desmostachya bipinnata, has been used as a diuretic and also to treat dysentery and menorrhagia, diarrhea, skin diseases and improving breast milk during lactation.

n. xi. Chandan, Santalum album, Sandalwood oil; has been widely used in folk medicine for treatment of common colds, bronchitis, skin disorders, heart ailments, general weakness, fever, infection of the urinary tract, inflammation of the mouth and pharynx, liver and gallbladder complaints etc.

n. xii. Sarala, Pinus roxburghii: Himalayan longleaf pine, Chir pine, Imodi pine, chir; resin exudate stimulant, internally stomachic, applied for insect bite, and skin affections; all parts of the plant are believed to possess medicinal qualities in Ayurveda. Chir pine is widely planted for timber & native to India. The turpentine is chiefly used as a solvent in pharmaceutical preparations, perfume industry, in manufacture of synthetic pine oil, disinfectants, insecticides and denaturants. The resin exudate is stimulant & internally stomachic; applied for insect bite, and skin affections externally. The alcoholic extract of the bark is used as antiseptic. The oil contains alpha pinene, longifolene and more terpene derivatives.

n. xiii. Kutaja, Psoralea corylifolia: Bakuchi, Somraji, Kushtananhini, Babchi, Bapunga, Bawuchee, Kalaginja, Bavanchalu are different names for this plant. The seed oil is also applied as a cure to leucoderma, contains psoralen and isopsoralin. It is used in the treatment of psoriasis; Somraji, in Charak Samhita or Bavanchalu have been used in the preparation made of rice.

It had profound effect on leprosy & skin diseases. Bakuchi seed powder with honey is useful in when taken internally and its oil/paste applied externally.

n. xiv. Kushta, Saussurea costus/S. lappa, Costus; the herb can tackle skin affections, used in asthma, cough, cholera, gout and rheumatism; root contains saussurine, and also bitter resin, root tonic, stomachic, carminative, stimulant, antispasmodic, exerts remarkable control in asthma and said to be used to cure even leprosy; It is a perennial herb, called kuth- & its roots are tonic.

It contains dehydrocostus lactone, costunolide and cynaropicrin which have anti-inflammatory & antitumor activities.

xv. Naga-Damani, Saussurea auriculata, Kushta, Kuth, Costus, Changalava cost, snow lotus, it is used in various traditional systems of medicine for its anti-ulcer, anti-

convulsant,anti-cancer, hepatoprotective, anti-arthritic, inflammation, skin healing with anti-viral activities. Changalava flower garland is said to be used by Lord Krishna.

n. xv. Point gourd, Trichosanthes dioica, Patola, Kommupotla, Patol, Patolam: Pointed gourd is a very ancient Ayurvedic medicinal herb and vegetable. It is used since the times of Charaka and Sushruta, >2000 years. It is very beneficial to improve gastric health.

Its root, leaf and fruit are used in many Ayurvedic medicines. Pointed gourd is told as a diet recipe for treating Kushta (skin diseases). It nourishes the liver and corrects all its functions. Working of the digestive system and the skin health are directly related with the working of liver.

Patola patra is a soft laxative detoxifies the body & cleanses the blood. Helps in maintaining healthy cholesterol limits and calms down the restless mind.

n.xvi. Eswaramooli, Arista-lochia indica, Hooka-bel, Ishwari,Isvaramuli, Esvaraveru, Dhumrapatra, Sunanda, Indian birthwort, Garudakkodi; it is a creeper; root tonic, stimulant, used in dry coughs, inflammation, & emetic in fevers; acts on nerves & the treatment of localized swelling. It can be fatal too as it restricts respiration in frogs and mice. Contains aristolochic acid, ceryl alcohol, and many more are present. It is a natural blood purifier.

The plant has been used in skin diseases. It is used as a appetizer, aphrodisiac and anthelmintic. The leaves and bark are used in bowel complaints of children, diarrhea and in intermittent fevers. In traditional medicine the underground parts of the plant are rubbed with honey and given to treat leprosy. Its leaves are macerated with black pepper as a prescribed in diarrhea. The root and stem of the plant are used in aches and pains, rheumatism, anthrax and madness. Juice of leaves used in snake bite. Its root is tonic, stimulant, emmenagogue and emetic. The roots are also used in fevers, and leukoderma. It contains aristolochic acid-D, aristolochic acid-D methyl ether lactam, aristolic acid and aristolic acid methyl ester etc.,

6.xviii.o. To avoid Injury, harden your skin. Atibala, Abutilon indicum, Kanghi, Paturi, Kangori, Tutturbenda, Panyara-ttuthi; Abutilon indicum- Infusion of leaves- demulcent, bark- astringent, diuretic, infusion of roots used in fevers; seed aphrodisiac, laxative, demulcent & used for removal of stones; Both root and bark diuretic, laxative, sedative, astringent, expectorant, anti-inflammatory. The oil made of the powder is said to be used as external body strengthener (atibala); the whole herb is used as demulcent, aphrodisiac, laxative, diuretic, sedative, astringent, and tonic.

The leaves showed the presence of amino acids, glucose, fructose and galactose. It contains abutilon A and more compounds. From the roots, non – drying oil consisting of various fatty acids viz. linoleic, oleic, stearic, palmitic, lauric, myristic, caprylic, capric and unusual fatty acids, is obtained. Sida rhombifolia is also called Atibala,-will be discussed in Sida species later.

Crack foot or Kurupulu or boils/wounds: Apply gorinta leaf paste on it or black jeera semi-roasted in ghee and applied as a paste or neem leaf paste applied to cure them.

O. ii. If injury is there: Tincture of iodine is the old way. Now people use betadine.

ii.a. The best is Achillea millefolium discussed at several places.

ii.b. Some more for wounds and ulcers best is Azadirachta indica: oil of its seed kernels showed antibacterial.

ii.c. Calotropis gigantea, (Sweta-arka) is active for topical application.

ii.d.Centella asiatica,-also known as mandookaparni, ii.e.haldi or Curcuma longa, ii.f.Lantana camara, g.gandana.

ii.h. Jatropha curcas used in the treatment of allergies, burns, cuts, wound inflammation, leprosy, leukoderma etc. ii.i.Strychnos nux vomica etc., is also useful.

ii.j.Aloe vera is also useful in wound healing as a diluent too. ii.k.Euphorbia neriifolia also good.

ii.l. Ficus racemosa is also good in injury healing.

O. iii. Mountain tobacco, Arnica Montana Flores, Leopard's bane, Mountain arnica, Wolf's bane, Arnica; rhizome and flowers-stimulant and sedative, injurious to frog and rat, leaf serve as poultice in swelling & bruises or pain, chapped lips and acne.

Arnica is applied for swelling associated with bruises, aches, sprains, and arthritis. It is used a sedative, bitter and even toxic. Its flowers are mild & cardiotonic. It is also applied to the skin for insect bite, muscle and cartilage pain, chapped lips, and acne. It is also taken by mouth for sore. Arnica may reduce swelling, decrease pain, and act as antibiotics. It has choline and betaine which contain adrenaline like activity with bruises, aches, sprains, and arthritis. It is used a sedative, bitter and even toxic. Its flowers are mild & cardiotonic. It is also applied to the skin for insect bite, muscle and cartilage pain, chapped lips, and acne.

and has a flavone that cause fall in blood pressure. It contains essential oils with thymol & flavanone glycosides. The flower heads constitute 0.2 – 0.8 % of Pseudo guaianolide sesquiterpenes;

o.iv. Brahma Kamal, Saussurea obvallata: The flower that Brahma was holding in hand is a white flower and hence called Brahma Kamal. It is of Saussurea obvallata. It is traditionally used for the treatment of paralysis, cerebral ischemia, wounds, cuts, bruises, liver disorders, bone-ache, cough, intestinal and urinal problems. The ground roots acts as a curative agent in wounds, pain, inflammation, boils, skin diseases.

o.v. The flower of Epiphyllum oxypetalum, Lady of the Night, Queen of the Night, Night blooming Cereus, Dutchman's-Pipe Cactus, Orchid cactus, which blooms at night is also said to be the Brahma Kamal, as it exactly looks similar. Epiphyllum oxypetalum is used in homeopathy and recommended for urinary tract infections, for heart conditions such as the crushing pain of angina and for spasmodic pain and haemorrhage.

The Brahma Kamal, the much-revered flower of the Himalayas, is an excellent example of plant life at the upper limit of high mountains (3,000-4,600 m).

o.vi. Ghamari, Bryophyllum pinnatum, Kalanchoe pinnata, Cathedral Bells, Zakham-e-Hyatt, Sima jamudu, Malaikalli, Pathar-chur, Patharchatta, Asthibhaksha- the roasted leaves are applied on boils/wounds/insect bites. Bryophyllum pinnatum is given for the treatment of a cough, asthma, cold with candy sugar. It is used against dysentery. The plant root is used to treat high blood pressure. It is also used to prevent any kind of cardiac problem. The herb is antiseptic, used in diarrhea, bruises, wounds, boils and even in insect bites. Its leaves are rich in malic and citric acids.

o.vii. insect bites:

i. Nisoth, Operculina turpethum, Pit-hari, Trivrt, Tellategada, Dudh-julmi, Tripula, Nisottar, (nisoth-means no cry), Indian jalap, white turpeth; Root and bark are cathartic and laxative. The tuberous roots are also efficacious cures fever caused by any of the tri-doshaa, stomach diseases, root used and prescribed in scorpion bite, gout, dropsy, melancholia, rheumatism, and even in paralysis; Trivrit causes purgation with root bark or leaves.-as powder 1-3 grams in divided dose per day. Its roots are purgative and prescribed in scorpion sting and snake-bite.

6.xix.p. Rheumatoid Arthritis

p.i. Here, if Janglipyaz, Urgenia indica, Urginea maritima-, Indian Squill, Vanapalandu,

Scilla indica (Baker), Ledebouria hyacinthina (Roth.), Nakka ulligadda- is added, it adds weight. These are used to treat joint pains the small bulbs diuretic, expectorant. it has scillarin-A and scillarin-B glycosides; cardiac stimulant.

It consists of the younger bulbs of Urginea indica (Knuth) and also known as diuretic, syrup and expectorant. Squill glycosides have cardiotonic properties. It is used in bronchial catarrh and it has scillaren A & B. It contains silli-glaucosidin has anti-cancer activity also. It yields small seed buds that are sold in Indian markets called gulchae, which contains garlic type compounds. So, garlic is also useful.

p. ii. Salai guggal, Boswellia serrata, Indian olibanum, Shallaki, Kunduru, Parangi sambrani; Indian olibanum gum is deodorant, diaphoretic, diuretic, astringent, emmenagogue, cures nervous diseases. Shallaki is used mainly for the treatment of osteo-arthritis and muscular pains. It is widely used as a substitute to modern pain killer medicines. It also is said to cure even cancer.

It is rich in boswellic acid, to be specific- four major pentacyclic-triterpenic acids i.e., β-boswellic acid, acetyl-β-boswellic acid, 11-keto-β-boswellic acid and acetyl-11-keto-β-boswellic acid. It relieves pain and improves joint mobility and flexibility. Indian sallaki is much more powerful than European olibanum in some cases.

It is also used for treating rheumatoid arthritis. It is indicated in treating asthma, ulcerative colitis, Crohn's disease etc. Its exudates are rich in boswellic acids & given as 1-3 g gum.

6.xx.q. Uterotonic: The best uterotonic is mango. However, depending upon the crisis, most frequently used herbs are Aloe vera, Abroma Augusta, Bambusa bambos, White Lotus or asoka (lodduga), Kumudam, Mullangi, papaya, Ficus species etc., Chemically uterotonics are papain or prostaglandin, Sesamin or ephedra species, vasicine or oxytocin or ergot alkaloids.

q. i. Juniper, Juniperus communis- fructus,- Common Juniper Hauber, Aaraar, Common Juniper, Dwarf Juniper, Hapusa; Common Juniper is a shrub; apply juniper oil directly to the skin for wounds and for pain in joints and muscles. Berry Carminative, stimulant, diuretic, useful in dropsy, leucorrhea, urino genital disorders;

q. ii. Lodduga, Symplocos racemosa, Symplocos paniculata, lodhra, Vellilathi, Vellilothram Lodhara, Lodhar, Pachotti, Mugam, Lodha, Symplocos *tree*, Asiatic Sweet-leaf; Medicinal Uses of lodhra is a tonic & emmenagogue; contain loturine and colloturine (harmine deriv); It is an evergreen Ayurvedic plant with anti-ulcer property. Powder of lodhra promotes wound healing with dhataki. Lodhra, nyagrodha bud, khadira, triphala and ghrta made into a paste provides looseness and softens hardened wound. Application of fine powder of lodhra twak promotes wound healing. It is also anti-HIV activity, with inhibitory activities against phospho-diesterase & anti-tumor too.

q. iii. Bala, Sida cordifolia: Indian ephedra, Country mallow, Gulipas, chiru benda, nil tutti, heart-leaf sida; Whole plant contains minor amounts of ephedrine and pseudoephedrine. Ephedrine is known to stimulate the central nervous system (CNS), and enhance weight loss; Its root decoction with ginger is febrifuge, its bark grinded or boiled inn sesame oil applied externally for facial paralysis. This herb is used to increase strength of body. Bala is an ancient Ayurvedic herb, used widely in a variety of Ayurvedic medicines. Its oil is to improve strength of bones, muscles and joints.

q. iv. Cohosh, Cimicifuga foetida, Sheng Ma, Bugbane, Pinyin,- native to Europe and Siberia, is used medicinally in China and India. Black Indian variety is Cimifoga racemosa, the previous herb. Chinese herb used in the treatment of prolapse of uterus and anus.

q.v. Ma-Huang, Ephedra geradiana, Ephedra, Asamania, Ain, Khanta, Buda-Gur, Chefrat, Somlata; Ma-Huang tincture is a cardiac & respiratory stimulant; decoction of roots and stem remedy for asthma, fever, difficulty in urination, rheumatism, even weakened cardiac muscles.

The tree produces fleshy, poisonous red cones which look like berries and juice of berries have capacity to improve respiratory passage; This herb is used as a peripheral vasoconstrictor, broncho-dilator and a central nervous stimulant. It is used for treating asthma, rheumatism, heart disorders and urinary disorders. It is diuretic and increases rate of perspiration. Its, herb & roots contain ephedrine and pseudo-ephedrine in 0.25-2.79%, along with flavonoids, lignans, catechols, polysaccharides, and tyrosine derivatives.

q.vi. American Ephedra, Ephedra trifurca, Log-leaf Mormon Tea, Longleaf Ephedra, Longleaf Joint fir, Mexican-tea, Mormon Tea, Ma Huang; used in China and USA many purposes like other species of ephedra. In China even injections are given in hospitals using these isolated products. Its pharmacological and medicinal uses are similar to Ephedra geradiana.

6.xxi.r. Some more Herbs with Disease Curative Property are given below

r.1.Urolithiasis or Stone in bladder or kidney: Kidney stone is a hard object that is made from chemicals of the type, calcium oxalate, uric acid, struvite, and cystine. Urinary tract stones begin to form in a kidney and may enlarge in a ureter or the bladder, most common for the consumers of muli, shalgam, kadam, etc vegetables with leaves as they are rich in oxalates. Kidney stones are also called renal calculi, nephrolithiasis or urolithiasis.

Tulasi is full of nutrients and is a remedy that has been used traditionally for digestive and inflammatory disorders. There are antioxidants and anti-inflammatory agents in basil juice, and it may help maintain kidney health. Basil contains Vitamin A, Vitamin K, Iron, Manganese, Calcium, and essential oils. Basil or tulasi contains eugenol, acetic acid, which helps break down the kidney stones and reduce pain.

The stones can also be reduced by using soanf, amla, tulasi, guduchi, Cynodon dactylon, but stronger are Caesalpinia nuga, Didymocarpus pedicellata, Berginia ligulata etc.,

r.2.Blood purifier: Salai guggal/Commophora Mukul, Curcuma longa, Hemidesmus indicus etc., Use fruits like apples, plums, pears and guavas have pectin fibre that is useful in cleansing blood. They not only bind with excess fats in your blood but also with heavy metals and other harmful chemicals or waste and remove them efficiently. The best way is to fast a day once a week.

r.3. Spleen enlargement: Cichorium intybus etc., Rohitak-arishta is an asava arishta spleen protective medicine in ayurveda. It is in for the treatment of enlarged spleen. Aphanamixis polystachya, the pithraj tree and also Rohitaka-Tecomella undulata are Ayurvedic herbs, used for the treatment of diabetes, jaundice, piles, intestinal worms, native to India- that work for spleen enlargement also.

r.4. Dropsy and urinary troubles: Cissampelos pareira, Gentiana kurro, Juniperus communis & Alfa-alfa (Medicago sativa) are suggested for use. When you pass large amounts of sodium in your urine that may result from foods you eat- causes a health problem for the kidney. Then, use of the herbs, like Haridra (Curcuma longa), Neem (Azadirachita indica), Shirish (Albizzia Lubeck), and Ashwagandha (Withania somnifera), or nim useful in recovery.

r.5. Eye diseases: Keep a clean muslin on eyes and put curd for half an hour and wash eyes. It works. The other herbs useful are Gingko Biloba (reduce glaucoma), Fennel (cures watery and inflamed eyes), Euphrasia rostkoviana *or* Eyebright, soothes itch and conjunctivitis.

r.6. Bowel complaints: Ginger: (digestive stimulant), Turmeric: (anti-inflammatory), Milk thistle (Silybum marianum- cures digestion), alfalfa etc.,

r.7. Tumor: Taxus baccata or Vinca rosea (sada-bahar) etc., but, use of inorganics in ayurvedic/unani also can make an early recovery. My own experience is that a suspected cancer (non-malignant) was eliminated by the use of mercury-based preparation, marketed as rasarath (Divya pharmacy) three Sachs, along with other medicines as recommended by an ayurvedic physician. All got eliminated completely. Read more in metals in ayurveda chapter for clarity.

6.xxii:s. Reducing a Poison: A Sudden Poisoning can be Handled by Age-Old Ways as below

s. i. Giving eranda oil about 50 ml so that all consumed foods are purgated with less absorption, or

s. ii. Give Madanphala (Randia dumetorum), to cause vomiting, or

s. iii. After any of the two above, give a about 5 to 10 grams of Sindhava salt. A drunken man is given salt solution as injection for recovery.

s. iv. Giving the extract of root of Ankotha (Alangium Salvi folium).

Even snake poison is a medicine. The solution to reduce poisons exist in many ayurvedic texts.

Here in general Cassia species in general serve as poison removers with good laxative properties. All Ficus species cure many diseases. Many Sida species are body toners and also fever curers. Modern medicines are good for spot relief, but with side effects like liver/kidney damage exist.

6.xxiii.t. Reducing Diseases

Further every Ficus specie serve as a good medicine. It is known those diabetics or some chronic disease patients- including cancer patients can find relief with herbal extracts, like tanged, and vempali. There are a number of plants; including the most important Kushta- can be used to dilute leprosy symptoms. Lord Krishna used to wear its flowers (cheti. lona. venna. chengalva. Poodanda")-means- butter in hand and garland of chengalva flowers (Naga Damani in Sanskrit is it Crinum asiaticum?). This herb finds use as Laxative, Purgative, Diaphoretic etc.,

See metals chapter where for more treatments discussed.

Some prefer elimination of disease through modern surgery, even I had two surgeries. But, the old ayurveda avoided surgery. That is the reason why most shunned use of ayurveda. No doubt some chronic diseases rarely get

eliminated. But, use of herbs can make the life smoother.

One example of treatment:

Tanged flowers dried (100gm), tanged seeds (10 gm), Cotton seed (50 gm), Dhania (50 gm.), Rose petals (20 gm), Sunthi (10gm), Chota-elachi (5gm),

Khas-khas (5gm) and Hemidesmus indicus (10 gm)-Such a mixture is made and stored and regularly consumed by putting @ 5gm, in boiled hot water. It is decanted within few minutes and extract consumed whole day. The extract lasts for three extractions or one day. Such a material with addition to shilajit can handle all poisons in about three months. Tangedu flowers are also used as vegetable. Here rela flowers (tanged) serve as a decoration for Batukamma festival and also as a vegetable too.

6.xxiv.u. Damaged Nerves

Each damaged nerve takes more than three months for replacement as there is no blood supply there. In case of paralysis, the part is nonfunctional as nerves are incapable of action, but the nerves communicate pain- there. Here giving the drugs like Rauwolfia serpentina roots help in the reduction of blood pressure. But, if there is some partial break/obstruction in the passage of blood in brain, it needs de-obstruent like glycerol for three or six months in small volumes along with medicines to clear it or present-day surgery does it. Here, the Indian use of garlic and ginger paste in foods never allow any nerve dysfunction. If there is impotency, it needs tonic like ashwagandha and also nerve activation using zinc or tin ions is also probably done. To clear earache, did you ever keep ear horizontally below water tap? Later, garlic oil insertion into ear, after cleaning it, seals its fate.

u. i. One of the best internal medicines recommended during the pakshaghata is garlic 4 grams thrice a day which generate fast degradation of proteins.

u. ii. Alternately, bala, atibala, guduci, sunthi, all mixed fine powders serve as tonics. (As 3-6 gm./day) – along with a laxative like Cassia fistula.

u. iii. To overcome exhaustion, the body is internally strengthened by bala (means strength, Sida cordifolia) as a tonic with guggal which act as analgesic-to treat internal nerve weaknesses.

u2. Strengthening Nerves

According to ayurveda, for survival one needs a strong body as it contains 340 joints and strong nerves through them. Activation of nerves can be done through anger or due to over-work or exercises or abuse-lead to exhaustion. A cool mind – eliminates such tensions. Further, the body is to be internally strengthened with bala (Sida cordifolia) as an internal tonic with guggal-to treat internal weaknesses. The body is externally strengthened by atibala and when it is applied externally as its prepared oil. This is said to be the Duryodhana's strength in Mahabharata. When my nerves and joints were with severe pain, I accepted all physicians suggested drugs for three years. I modified this treatment through external application of honey- once a day on joints-for six months. However, nervous disorder can be handled with herbs like Abrus precatorius, Acorus calamus, Curcuma longa, Nardostachys jatamansi, Centella asiatica etc.,

6.xxv:v. Drug Resistance

When an infection strikes, only modern medicine exists. In the recent times the antibiotic resistance is common in many patients. How to counter such resistance? The simplest aspect is using plant or ayurvedic or unani drugs as they have less drug resistance from bacilli. Further, using multiple herbs can even destroy it or dilute it.

6.xxvi.w. Herb Adulteration

The next problem is about medicinal herb adulteration. This adulteration can be due to several reasons. The herbal adulteration in a simple way can be categorized at least into four varieties.

A. The basic herb is available in plenty and not properly collected at the right time.

B. If the selected plant material is not available in large amounts, replacement is done with an equivalent material of genuine grade. This led to imports.

C. But a deliberate substitution with equivalent amounts with another material; or with inferior/cheaper substitutes. Another example is Mustard seeds mixed with aalia seeds;

D. The next mustard seeds during oil preparation, a deliberate addition of Argemone Mexicana seeds for pungency.

E. Commercial handling of the plant material leading to another specie addition. eg. Punarnava is mixed with punarnavi, where one herb is active and the other is not.

In conclusion, my discussion on health ends here. Most details are suggestive in nature. Only diseases common & useful in my opinion – are covered & many diseases not mentioned.

However, in extreme cases like hospitalization, which needs a physician-not discussed here. For more refer Charak Samhita/any authentic text/physician.

These are the visible details and hence marked as SAT (sat means truth/visible in my opinion). Most details are suggestive in nature.

But, coming subjects are only an explanation to the impacts received by the body as one can see nothing, through a normal eye. What are they?

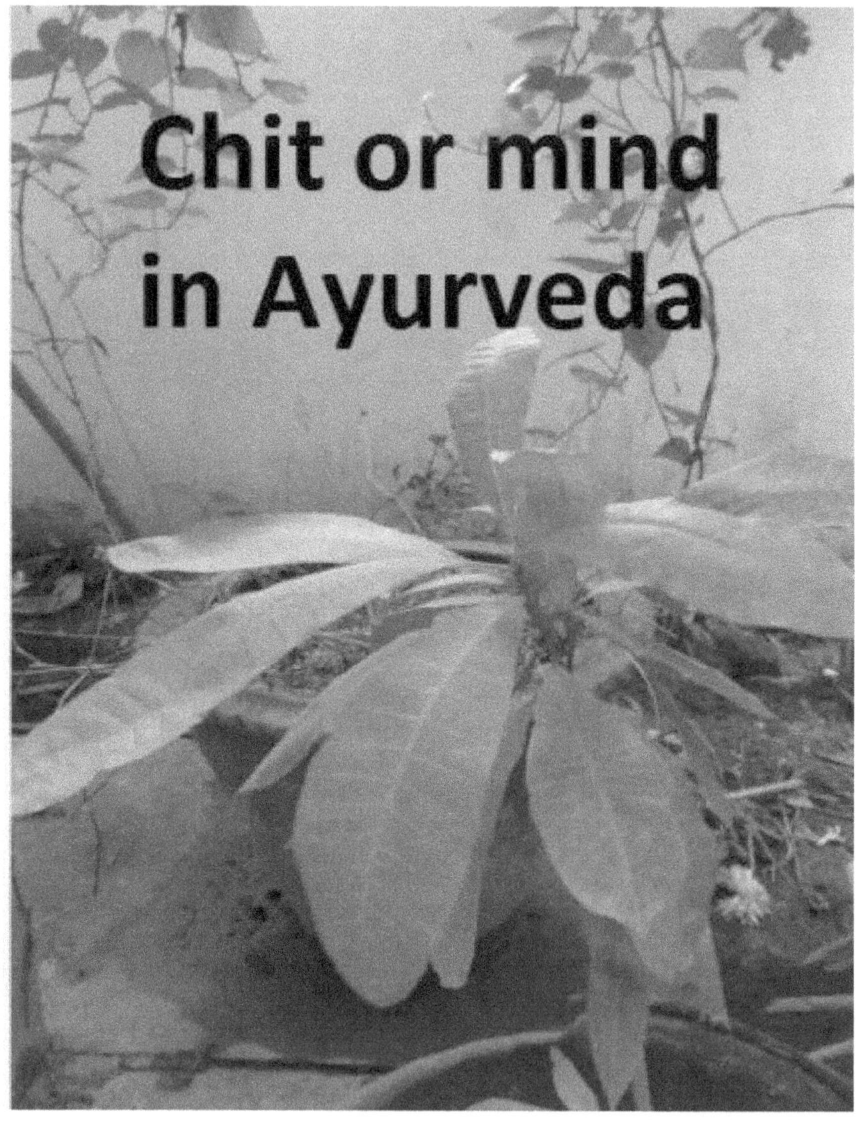

Cashew plant

Part - III

Chit - The Invisible Factors Affecting Health

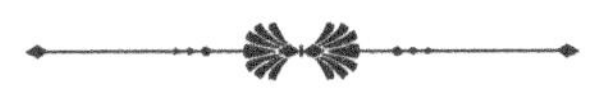

7. Ayurvedic Theory (Simplified)

The invisible effects on our body need to be understood (Sushruta samhita) without which, the subject of health is incomplete. A person is declared dead when his brain is non-functional (Chaitanya is not there or chit/soul is lost).

What is chit? The chit can be either soul/mind/a person's consciousness- depending upon the place where it is used. Impact on mind is only a felt due to the unseen impacts. The theory of ayurveda is also an explanation to these invisibles.

Theory: All worldly creations according to the theory, fall into four categories; namely-Jarayuja – animals including mammals; Andaja- egg born creatures (animals); Swedaja-filth born worms and insects; Udbhijja- trees, shrubs etc.,

i. Body & panca-mahaboot: Coming to the humans – all fall into the category of jarayuja and are made up panca- mahaboot-s; namely- Prithvi- that makes the whole body; Akash- for medhas – Brain/mind; Vayu – chest; Tejas – Stomach; Jala – Liver and lower parts; Out of the panca-mahabhoot, even if one is missing, the person is dead.

But, the panca-mahabhoot actually exist outside the body. Sun and moon are a part of Brahmandam (Universe) and our body is a pindandam – that is in Lainson with panca-mahabhoot. This is the basic theory. In namaskar mudra-our soul is saluting its counter parts through Idol.

"Man is above animal because he is gifted with speech, expression & intellect. Only he can do good or bad to the nature or society-whereas animals work only for their survival and also help man in his survival as he is superior."

7.ii: Asta chakra nava dwarah-: In another sloka-: "Asta-chakra-Nava- dwarah- dehanam- purah- ayodhya"-means- The body so formed is controlled by eight energy centers (asta chakra). Further it had nine entries cum outlets like a village-making body-an ayodhya or no war zone. The present Ajodhya is symbolic of India's soul is another dimension, la soul to the body!

Stomach generates energy from food and distributes energy through blood. When the energy reaches all parts of the body a beaming face emerges. The birth of man is revealed in purusha-suktam. But, where are these chakras?

Visuddha and four finger widths to above be ajna chakra and two finger width to above is Sahasrara (brain) through the spinal cord.

Spinal cord: Surprisingly these chakras are positioned exactly opposite to the other in the spinal cord. There are three chakras-below are- probably expanded from DNA of a woman- (as- @2" width, @ 3" width & later@ 9") that hybridizes with man's DNA as

(@9", @3" and @2"-) to become, another three chakras- supplied from above.

Heart: Thus, the heart and its begins with mooladhara, from the base of spinal cord as the first chakra. Its above-after two finger width is next chakra- called swadhistana. The next above with four finger width (Betha) on spinal cord is manipurak, (the third chakra. Again, above one jaana to above is Anahata chakra. From there to above one jaana is lungs form-fusion point of two expanded DNAs-that form Anahata chakra. This heart has 101 nevers near or around it that controls its beats.

Eighth chakra: Since only seven chakras are accounted, where is the eighth chakra?- it is said to be controlled by the entrapped soul in the heart and it has a unique path through sushumna naadi to the top. It is the last chakra-called aura or some call it as Niralamba, or non-inclined attached to the delicate point in the Centre of skull – called maadu or brahma-randhra (Telugu). It is through that our soul can either escape or communicate with the parent or the almighty.

7.iii. Dosha: Ayurveda further proceeds in three parts, namely-preservation, promotion, eliminate or restrict diseases for survival. Our survival is due to good skin which prevent diseases. Even the skin thickness in man- is directly proportional to the thickness of the grain – called vriha (at the Gujarat Ayurvedic University, Jamnagar 1984) – as given in Sanskrit sloka.

What one can see is that-a person wakes up before sunrise,-called pradosha kaal (prior to dosha period). Hence, it means, no activity is no dosha. But food is a necessity-on which-all living organism depend upon and it is the first dosha.

But, how to define a dosha?

Dosha is disease or in other words dis---ease or un-easiness- can be due to physical or mental sickness. The physical sickness can be diagnosed as Vata, Pitta/& Kapha or their combinations.

7.iv. Kapha, Pitta &Vata:

Vata dosha can be due to the problem generated to the free movement of air- which is external. Bur respiration is a must for survival and it is the-Prana Vayu- that reaches- brain and lungs. Udaan Vayu (Umbilicus, chest and throat), Samana Vayu as Supply to digestive juices; Vyana Vayu – waste accumulated through blood circulation and partly released as Apana Vayu through intestines.

The process of crushing the food (pit – ga-ya – is pitta) in the stomach and further in the intestines.

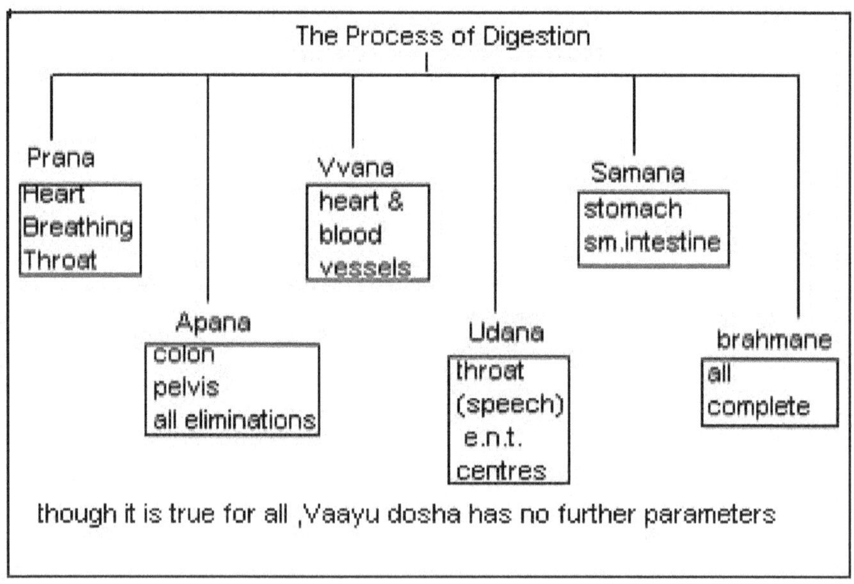

How it acts? Ranjaka in liver and spleen; Bhrajaka- to provide skin, pigments, hair etc; Alocaka- to provide vision and thinking; Sadhaka- provides intelligence and ego with sadhana (experience).

So, kapha and pitta act together to crush food and they are aided by (vata) oxygen through lungs.

Kapha means sleshma which can be of five variations. Its close word is cough, which comes with abnormality in solid food consumed. Viz., Kledaka- situated in stomach, to moisten food & provide protection to the walls of digestive organs from being hurt; Avalambaka-provide nutrition to heart; Tarpaka-provide nutrition to brain; Bodhaka – recognition of taste-associated to our intellect or buddhi; Slesaka is to lubricate all joints.

This is my simple way of understanding this subject & most of the times – an overloaded stomach leads to kapha; highly protein and oil rich food consumption leads to pitta and finally raw meat/salads/unclean water etc., can lead to vata (fungal) diseases.

There is no hardliner demarcation among vata, pitta and kapha, but for detection purposes, these terms are still in use. Here, fasting is an important way of treating the body.

A chess player comes with fresh mind & almost with empty stomach and takes lemon juice after the play. An injured deer or dog fasts and sleeps in a hideout/in a bush-till recovery.

7.v: Identification of a disease: According to my understanding of ayurvedic terms, one is hungry, thirsty, suffering with headache or sprain; saw some horror scenes etc., it is an impact felt by the body. Similarly, many abnormalities are invisible (avykta) & not seen by a physician.

Likewise, attack on the body through bacilli is not visible to the naked eye, but locatable through its expression. But there are some diseases that need time for proliferation-like infection, jaundice, typhoid, tuberculosis etc., which remain dormant (sushupta) for a long time.

But some diseases rapidly express like fever, diarrhea, injury etc.,- (Vyatka) visible and physician responds with immediate attention.

From the physician's view point- all are dosha and all need an immediate attention. The physician diagnoses any disease as kapha, pitta, Vayu or their combinations.

If the disease is severe in nature, a physician is called for diagnosis. Then, he looks into many other factors- as in sloka-

"Niidanam…. Puurva… roupaani… roupahsyu – paraayasta-tha- samprapti-shyo-scheti vijnanam… roga-naam. … Pascha-tha – srutamu"

That means, when a disease is struck, the physician looks into these factors for a solution, by sitting in vimana (plane) stana.

What are they? It is the manifested symptoms or indications with exploratory observations give knowledge to detect the disease. What observations are to be made then? Nadi (pulse); mutra (urine); mala (feaces); jihva (tongue); sparsha (touch); caksu (eye); akriti (shape).

This is what modern physician also is doing. But now physician adds more expensive tests!

7.vi: Agni/Tejas/Fire: If there is a short fall of Agni in the body, result is ama – with semi-digested food or body becomes mala sanchaya. So, either bhutagni or dhavagni is in short supply. Fasting is also termed as "Lan-khanam param-oushadham"- but with caution towards some disease born/pregnant/old/injured etc.,

The process of formation of Agni in Indian philosophy-is made of three modes of fire. If all subdivisions are looked into, this Agni is further subdivided into thirteen variations. The vital one is jatharagni or hunger. The next being the sapta-dhatu- Agni-inside the body-generated through enzymes- all summed up to make thirteen Agni.

The enzymatic digestion is also termed as Agni. The eyes have the capacity to see, order and also guided by ajna-chakra. The mouth has the capacity to release Agni through strong words- using air and mind-in the form decisive actions. Body is ever heated to maintain at 98.4°F which is again Agni.

The invisible- molecular level is sapta-dhatu-Agni. Thus, adenosine triphosphate (ATP) or NADPH or any enzyme(s) etc., are also dhatu-Agni.

Finally, it is our integration with nature (panca-mahabhoot-s) provide panca-bhutagni like home, wood, water, fire & air and finally food. Basically Agni means tejas – it comes through digestion of food in the stomach. It is called – jatharagni, & other enzymes supplement this agni.

7.vii. Dushya: Excreted/rejected part is dushya. If fasting is ignored or over-eating done, the net-result is dushya (undigested/un-excreted). It gets excreted in nine types modes – sveda- (sweat); nakha-(nails); kesa-(hair); stanya – (milk); sukra – (semen); ansu-(tears); mala & mutra- (feaces and urine); spota- (solid rejections through skin); svasa-(respiration). If any process fails, dushya exists in the body. A well-fed rat is always lies sleeping and a starved rat is active in search of food. So, dushya is a problem that comes with indigestion/non-elimination of digested stuff in time.

7.viii. Ayurveda has lot of focus on mental faculty. How this mind or chit can be manipulated?-using a concept of philosophical mind and God. Leave all problems to Guru or God and they disperse your problems systematically.

The next question- why the problems arise?- according to the scholars, it is your past karma is the reason for birth & present deeds add to karma or sin or their reduction.

Thus, an average individual is given a good adaptable path for survival, with peace of mind. It is here, religion plays important role. What are the factors that play with mind?

Mind and food: Here, food is essential for survival. Can food affect our mind? (The answer can be yes or no). How ayurveda in good old days studied the impact of food? Here, even fasting is an important way of remembering the God. Fasting restricts- the crime rate and it also clears clogged GI Tract to normalcy.

Fasting also gives sometimes a clean thought or clear vision. Thus, devta (angel) work with a sattvic mind and share some traits of the creator.

Sattvic mind: Indra (symbol of authority and Lordship & farsightedness) or Yama (observe the propriety of actions and initiate right action in time) or Varuna (have patience and dislike impurity, he is also brave & exhibit anger) or Kauvera (kuber is fond of money & possessive) or Gandharva (fond of dance and singing & enjoy praise and music). or sanyasi/saint/Yogi, or Rishi/a pure and pious soul- who broke from family & traditions/stopped indulging are followers of the path of Lord Shiva – can be any of the three-but termed sattvic by me.

The life is not that smooth as it seems to be. So, it creates more traits in the brain that cause passion, anger, greed, ego, ignorance, jealousy, dejection or intolerance etc., these thoughts can be with Rajasic or tamasic minds.

Rajasic mind: A rajasic mind carries with it a huge tradition like kings. Hence their mind has capacity to add more mental traits with continuous rajasic foods,- to a different level, Asura, Pai Sacha, Sarpa, Rakshasa, Praita, or Shakina types.

Thus, he develops pick and choose methods. This is not the end. Still there is a scope to manipulate a mind and this leads to another group that is tamasic.

Tamasic mind: There exists another mind that comes out of dejection or manipulative suppression within the society. Such a mind adds more traits as below.

Pasava (selfish or like animal), Or Masya (suspicious or fishy in attitude), Or Vavnaspatay (wavering & fecal mind) etc.,

Thus, there are different types of persons with mental variability- sub-grouped as sattvic, rajasic and tamasic.

Thus, person's food can alter or bring changes his or her mental attitude in a conclusive way. Here Lord Krishna added more points- like how you earned your living also imparts the living. For example, eat chilies to get anger is a proverb. If one goes through 14th, 16th &17th chapters in Bhagavad-Gita, the impact of food, difference between devta (angel) and asura (demon)- all were elaborated by Lord Krishna himself.

7.ix: Sapta dhatu: The function of sapta-dhatus need to be understood. What are they?

Rasa: Rasa leads to internal digestion and adsorption of food and the failure of which leads to diseases like, asradha (anorexia), aruci (distaste), asyavairasya (bad taste in the mouth), asasajnata (ageusia).

Rakta: Rakta is the carrier of all diseases as it touches all parts of the body and its weakness can lead to every type of disease starting from fever, jaundice etc.,- as it is a carrier.

Mamsa: the bones and muscle are strengthened through soft portion of muscle, mamsa, but get accumulated through rakta.

Medas: Medas, the vital centre of all nerve functions also has an excretory process of hair, burning sensation of body, dryness of mouth & throat etc.

Asthi: Bones, their formation & growth, bone fractures etc.,

Majja: Pain in the finger joints, giddiness (bhrama), fainting (murcha), and lameness due to abscess of the joints.

Sukra: Lack of sukra or its vitality can lead to sterility, or impotency, deformation in offspring etc.

Here, one finds that the minerals are capable of meddling to influence dhatu. Dhatu is derived from dharana which means to hold & dhatu can also be a metal.

In the chapter on metal use in ayurveda many minerals-essential-were discussed already. The people wear multi metal rings, kada etc.

The body also has some upa-dhatus like, kandara, shira, vasa, tvak, etc.- making it a complex mechanism to understand.

Taste: Ayurvedics describe the drug effects through rasa(taste), Roopa (look/appearance), gandha- (odor)-like tikta (bitter),

Kashaya (astringent), Madhura (sweet) and also Guna (attributes like laghu (light), ushna (hot) etc.), prabhava (therapeutic effects), viipaka (resultant or after effects): virya (potency). The practice of ashtanga way- of treatment is known since Mahabharat (chapter 5-sloka 93). Even today, there are books on astanga-hridaya.

A condensed version of theory related to the food is in Bhagavat Gita & also deals with mind. Saint/rishi/yogi/sanyasi (renunciatory) is above all, yet are sattvic.

Thus, mind can have multiple traits- which are associated to food and also circumstances. So, we have already entered into the subject mind.

According to Santana dharma (cosmic Law), our every action is being noted by the nature, but with no visible sign to a commoner. There is a need to discuss invisibles. Nature tolerates harmonious actions and uneven deeds can retaliate at some stage.

8. Chit / & Mind

If the, mind can have multiple traits. But what is mind and where it is? Can you see it?

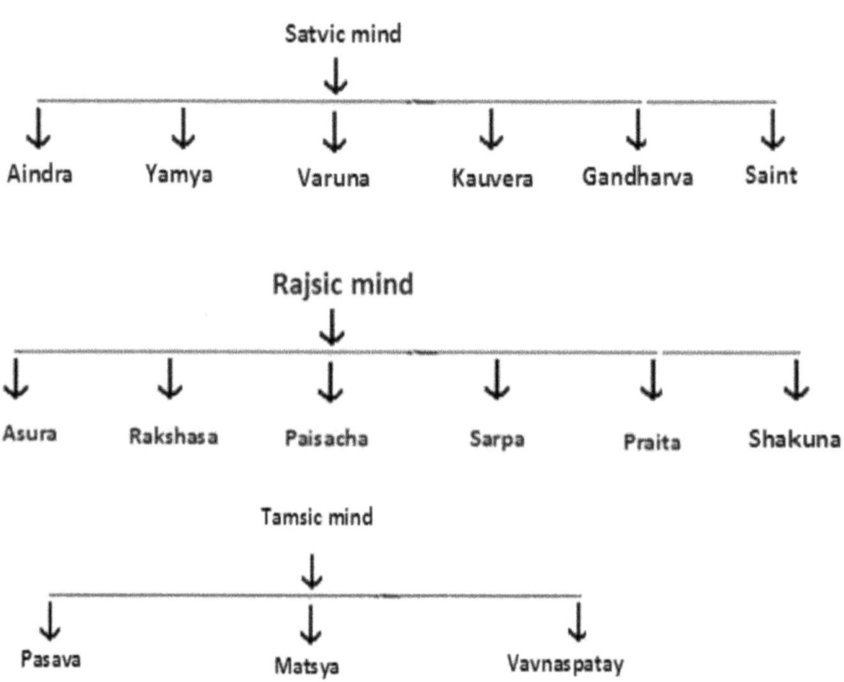

8.i. Nature: In the previous chapter, the impact of food on the mental trait is well explained. But the body has many functions in it with five types of recognitions (panca-jnan-endriya)- Sabda, Sparsa, Rasa, Roopa, Gandha, (hear, touch, taste, look & smell). Similarly, there are also six evils- Kama (desire), krodha (anger), lobha (greed), moha (passion), mada- matsarya-(money or power associated deeds) – all are associated with the body but they impact our mind. They get associated with the new born from the nature and they end with the body-after the soul flees.

8.ii. Mind and intellect: We have already studied the impact of food vis-a vis mind. If one considers mind as the source of thinking, and action, it is guided by buddhi- means all three exists in our body.

Chit: What more the scriptures suggest? Chit is a Sanskrit word that can have multiple meanings. Coming to us, chit can be our mind or soul or consciousness. Mann, Buddhi, Chit, Ahankara is separately mentioned, where chit is consciousness. Most of the time chit means mind.

8.iii. Mind & Greed: Similarly, the scholars have put greed the tree of sins- (lobha. ha. papasya… kaaranam) – responsible for all miseries. The tree of lobha is shadowed by another force maya (money/desires). Thus, it is lobha that incites to wrong actions through poisoning of mind. Then, anger gets attached- leading to buddhi-bhrasta (loss of wisdom). This leads to kuta- neethi (dark/ shaded actions) & kshudra (dirty deeds).

The end result is a misery and mental disturbance. This needs mental coolants for sleep and for all troubles, sleep is the best medicine. Thus, mind is the most critical part of the brain that can make/break our health.

8.iv. Mind &Yoga: There are many sloka-s, but I mention two related to yoga, "yogaescha. chitta. vritti. nirodhaha." And another "Dharana…s.cha…yogyataa… Manasseh". So, it is possible to restrict wavering of mind and also can be controlled through pranayama (respiration) & practice.

8.v. Mind & Harmony: Mind is the mental-oscilloscope of an individual that interacts with buddhi (wisdom) and the entrapped soul. Thus, we have all three – namely, soul (spirit), chit (mind) and buddhi (wisdom or intellect)- exist in our body & they ought to have a harmonious relationship for all good actions.

If the mind is in your control, you can be called Rudra (powerful Shiva) and if it oscillates with desires, one behaves like Lord Indra-who is known to succumb for every desire. An average man is a variant between these two extremes. But all such actions need a strong network of nerves.

The nerves arethe communicative lifeline of the body, through which the sorrow or happiness or anger or any feeling- reaches the brain & soul. Indian philosophy suggested that there are 72,000 nerves in a human body. They get supply from eda, pingala (input & output) – nadir-vyavasta. The scriptures indicate the presence of another-sushumna naadi that is the third mode of communications through nerves in the body. For example, the heart- weighing less than a kg.- is surrounded by approximately 101 nerves- is the theory.

Here anger destroys or burns your nerves. If one remains cool (thand..rakh) nerves remain intact – without damage. There are several aspects in strengthening the nerves thereby increasing immunity.

8.vii. Nastik/Aethist: According to a hetuvada or nastic/atheist, man by himself is responsible to his deeds! For him, with no faith in God- mental coolants are a needed to prevent its volatility in mind-like somras (alcohol) or nalla-mandu (opium)/hallucinogens. Now, several new psychotropic drugs entered the market-thanks to scientific inventions.

Astik: In the initial stages, a deep faith on guru – brings-in a cool mind for an astik (with deep faith in God)- gets peace by surrender to God/guru. In order to make positive impact on mind- precious stones/ornaments/kada/rudhraksh/even herbal pacifications/faith-cure/fasting/wearing animal objects on hand or neck etc.-are well known.

8.viii. Renunciation: Another way is that- to disengage mind from worldly desires – a procedure called renunciation (sanyas),-that brings a peace of mind. This elevates the mind & opens the Pandora box of mysteries. A positive mind leads to acquisition of magic or siddhi (acquisition of powers).

8.ix: Body, mind and Environment: According to Dev Prasad Sahu, an ayurveda practitioner, "The basic concept of disease is a manifestation of consequences of the interplay between body, mind and the environment which creates a difficult dilemma for the physicians & medical scientists".

Next problem is that if your neighborhood colony is not clean, can you anticipate a good health? Thence, the human body is in balanced state only when all five mahabhut-s are in appropriate proportion- which means, physical & mental cleanliness, and also clean environment.

8.x. Body, and Atman (soul): What is a soul? – it is difficult to answer. The body has a soul that brings in Chetana (activity) to the body. If someone is capturing or seizing your mind/brain, making it immobile, one has no choice except to consult an expert-who understands the invisible or something above the body. It is beyond our five senses. That means there is a direct communication between soul (atman) & mind.

Lord Krishna declared that atman is indivisible. Once there was a study to know the difference between live and the dead- by keeping a dying person on a balance type bed. But its difference was negligible or practically immeasurable.

Thus, atman with an insignificant weight-forces movement in a huge body that weighs from two kilos up to 200 kilos or even more.

It orders the body to move & even run and it runs. But, when the soul quits, the body needs at least four persons to lift it!

For an atheist fusion of DNAs is leading to entrapped air- is the new off-spring- or new soul.

8.xi. Third eye: There is a barrier which a normal person cannot cross. Thus, it brings-in the concept of another dimension or third eye which Lord Shiva- is known to possess and he is called Bhootnath (leader of devils). He only he can foresee the incoming trouble.

If some good soul exists, there is every possibility that troubled souls also exist. It is here, tantric (Bhoota- Vaidya) who look for troubled souls and help in their solace. But, without the body, there is no expression for any soul.

8.xii: Mind and God: The first visible god is the Sun (more in astrology). Stanza in Sanskrit deals with most aspects connected to life in man. It suggests- "chandrama, manaso—jaatah. Chaksho. Surya." It means mind is controlled by moon; eyes contain Tejas (fire)…" The criterion of life can be an entrapped air or ether- called atman (As in purustasuktam, 'Prana.t…Vayu.Rachayata'- in both Telugu and Sanskrit- referring to the spirit/soul).

Then where is God?

The scriptures indicate the following.

A. First hint- "peeta – bhas-wa-ty—anu—samah" means-an anu (atom size) yellowish shining Sun is visualized in our body.

B. Finally, where?-It is a place-

("naabhayam...upari. Tishtathi")- from umbilicus to above by one jaana or @9"-and also below visuddha chakra again by one jaana--- means in the heart.

C. How he is present?- "-sa-Brahma.... Siva.... Hari.sya- Indra. paramo.... smaraat"- it means —God (or Guru) is found along with Brahma, Shiva, Hari, Indra,-- or whom one prays as God is in his own heart!

8.xiii. Re-birth: It is said that there is a neutral matter-called Bramham (or God)-much above us. If any soul reaches there it is bliss or moksha or free from rebirth. But, in general, there are many souls floating around Bramham-with desires and are waiting to take re-birth at appropriate time. Thus, faith is individual aspect.

Further, God/soul exist in everyone and all humans are a precious creation of his parents. The more one goes through such sloka, the more he gains the subject!

8.xiv: Mind & Religion: How religion acts?- It is true that every religion guides our travel from darkness to light. Every religion suggests a specific adoptable path or procedure for a peaceful living or to reach salvation or God. So, mind can be baked to militancy or can be cured to be peaceful through religious philosophy. A religion is guided by the circumstances. According to the Bible, when Jesus resurrected himself- after crucifixion or after the so-called death. Then people doubted his version. Then Jesus ordered Lazarus to come out and Lazarus broke his coffin & came out alive with a beaming smile. That was the capacity of Jesus Christ- that he can recreate!

Thus, an innocent Adam & Eve, created by God- ate for-bidden fruit & started gaining knowledge and rose to the highest level – like Lord Krishna. Thus, we have no balances & to measure the capacities of these stalwarts or Saints or even an individual's faith in God.

Lord Krishna suggested that – just as- we remove old torn clothes to acquire new dress; the soul also changes the body-through death (chapter2-22nd sloka in Bhagavat Gita). There are persons even today, capable of reading through the finger print-to give details of the previous birth.

In Australia, some modern experiments with tape recorders – are said to have been done to understand the whispers of the weeping souls or the dead errant souls. It means there is a search for new modes- to decipher grievances of a soul – which so far is a Tantrika's monopoly.

8.xv. Mind & Myth: Renunciation is the first step towards the eternal world. If one practices more on mind one can be a magician Mandrake or P.C. Sarkar, about whom, I heard. But I have seen Bhagavan Satya Sai Baba producing objects & vibhuti (ash) from empty hand. Even late Sri Krishna Jyothi Shi (Jammu Maharaj) whom I met several times, was a miracle man. This comes with their long practice on mind- called tapas.

8.xvi. Capacity of mind: According to Jaggy Vasudev (religious guru), one can divert his mind even in ten different directions at a time and still, it can come up with answers for every direction. That is the capacity of mind. I am a witness- to have seen asta- avadhanam in "The Hindu college, Machilipatnam (A.P) in @1970". The author was posed eight different questions by scholars and he came up with answers as well-versed poetic stanzas in about two and half hours-along with gossip!

Bhagavan Sri Satya Sai Baba's discourses were simple and informative. I have attended to such discourses in Puttaparti. His discourse used to draw inspiration from Quran, Bible or Taoism and his representation of lamp (Jyoti) which is surrounded by symbols of all major religions. He was also a miracle man, who cured many.

8.xvii. Philosophy: Philosophy is also essential for peaceful living/salvation and it begins with renunciation. You cannot always win with might. Thus, one should be philosophical to pardon the errant.

Shirdi Sai Baba told his devotees to leave problems to him and do their duties in peace of mind. He even helped or answered their problems from grave. The vital question is that how to come out of mental tension?

The mantra suggests," sahanam. bhavatuh…"- means show tolerance. Here, in Hindi the saying goes" thand. rakh." – be cool in crisis even if something is wrong.

8.xviii: Woman and Yuga dharma: All Yuga-s are guided by four stalwarts, namely Shiva (Krita Yuga), Rama (Treta Yuga), and Krishna (Dvapara yuga) and Durga (Kali Yuga). Why man lost his powers and how a woman gained? –

According to Manu-the first creator of humans, "Na-stree. Swatantra. yam. Arhati"- a woman do not deserve independence and it was observed true as it suited man and his might. Where is the woman later? She did not fight in Krita-yuga or Treta-yuga, or Dvapara-yuga and even now-unless compelled.

She was even diced like a commodity in Dvapara-yuga. The net result is the war of Mahabharat – that killed and uprooted the errant. This is because; man ruled/still ruling- Nature/& woman by force. Zarr-zoru-zamin or three wine- women-wealth which man still wish to control.

Man forgot the saying, "Raamoh.Vigrah. Vann. Dharma." – means Rama or every action of Rama is according to dharma. The subsequent rulers forgot Rama's basic rule 'mana. Vaak. Karmanah'…. meaning practice that rule which you think, practice and follow.

Later rulers subverted the rules by saying 'the rules are for fools. Thus, with each Yuga, animal man-with four legs- lost one leg in each yuga and now the final is Kaliyuga with the man is with one leg- means became immobile. Man's real/ate is well depicted by Lord Jagannath of Puri (Odisha) as a statue with no hands or legs.

Hence, woman gained all powers by serving man and thus mother/Durga is depicted with all weapons!

Woman is-Om prakriti-y-namah in Lakshmi stotram or nature-deciphers action in a congenial way. Thus, Nature or Prakriti or Viswam or Universe- are different names proposed for an elevated woman. When, man visualized the real strength of nature and he wrote Sri-Suk-tam.

Hence, Shiva parted a half of his body to his wife, Vishnu kept his wife in his chest and Brahma kept his wife on his tongue. This is because, 'Viswame. Veda. Purusha-stha-viswam-. upah. jeevathi' (Purushasuktam in Telugu).- means the entire universe is a Veda (unchallengeable truth),- wherein man (purusha is closer to parusha which means a ruffian) – has to live in harmony with the Nature- lest he can

lose the co-existence prematurely- leading to nature's fury through calamities.

So, Prakriti is conservative & in its or her opinion. But Purusha is explosive and he forces his opinion. Unless he is explosive, can he land man on moon? Then, why man is adamant?- It is like a widely grown tree or shrub is trimmed or shaped by a Gardner. The same way, man or woman- need pruning by a guru. Thus, guru suggests & others implement action and hence, it is a co-existence for survival.

If one visualizes man as a discovering scientist, & woman as an experienced technologist, their combination is science & technology- which can give a patented expression or new off-spring.

8.xix. Insomnia/sleeplessness, the problems and the consequences: Sleeplessness is a most common problem that existed with humans since their birth. All other animals peacefully sleep and have no such problems. Why? It is because they have nothing to hide or nothing to stake to lose only survival is the motto. But for humans, the desires are peculiar as they shadow the opponent and kill if possible as a revenge and it leads to sleeplessness. Thus, root cause is somewhere else.

For example, a person is in deep forest and it is infested with wolves, tigers, and snakes etc., So, he cannot afford to sleep. Even during Ramayan, the king Dasarath was sleepless as he gave two boons to his wife Kaikeye. Thus, sleeplessness was associated with power and money.

Later, during the end of war of Mahabharata, the teacher Drona's son, Ashwatthama gave more reasons for sleeplessness and added more points for it. He said the people who accumulated lot of wealth (legal or illegal), one who is fond of free sex, and the third is beware of most harmed as they are ought to be revengeful. For example, general Vaidya of India was murdered even after his retirement and another example is collapse of twin towers in USA. Thus, though the quotes were old, the results are visible.

Final, Sant Kabir said" boya ped babool, aam kaheko hoye"

According to a modern boss,- extracting boons like Dashrath of Ramayana- says that the rules are for fools and free to do every damage in the name of jurisdiction. A live testimony is the chief sculptor of Konark temple, during construction, failed to complete his work, another young sculptor came and completed it. The chief felt insulted, then went and murdered him in the same temple. The dying person yelled,-o, father, I am your lost son! It is a temple where no meditation – a live testimony of revengeful consequences- bloodletting.

The golden rule is that – work hard to the best of your ability and you are assured of good sleep. A hard-working laborer always has deep sleep on the roadside or on sand deserts. This is done by Ram (Ram stayed in parnashala in the forest), Lakshman, hanuman, and even pandava brothers were in forests. Pandavas have been hidden in a cave, which looks like a hill (a hole covered with stone). It still exists in Gujarat. The cave had two rooms and can be closed by a good stone and their presence remain un-noticed.

8.xx. Kaal chakra: The kaal-chakra begins- with the new born. kaal-chakra begins to count your number of breaths from the birth & to terminate your life- kaal- acts as soon as the count is complete. It is like reverse count for a rocket release, the soul flees from the body.

The faster is the respiration, the early is the death. See dog (18 years, > 6 respirations/minute) to tortoise (400 years- one respiration/4 minutes) and man is in the middle. A Yogi can reduce or stop breathing-to prolong his life.

Every saint has the capacity to break kaal-chakra. Lord Shiva is the true symbol- a yogi-raja, who broke the kaal-chakra (time). The beauty lays with an elevated soul as it can come back into the body &

can reactivate life. Thus, Shiva, resurrected himself at several places in India- including his meeting Adi-shankara and their discussion is in the form of five questions by Lord Shiva (Manisha- pancakam).

So, Lord Shiva-as an Idol- is ever watching & listening (drusyatae & sruyatae)- a feat, that is not simple. Adi-Shankara, in order to answer a query, left his body, noted the facts and resurrected himself – nearly after about a month-to reply Bhatruhari's wife's query!

Hence, Yogi's body is buried as it responds to your problems. A saint's capacity is not susceptible to any type of measurements.

Here the sayings like- fear of God is the beginning of wisdom- or "Parvat-nigar-alam"- exist- all to correct an errant. Mahatma Gandhi

proposed- do not see bad- do not talk bad- do not think bad referring to the three monkeys of the mind.

For peace of mind, Bhagavan Satya Sai baba suggested- to keep a ceiling on one's own desires- as first step to restrict mind. Here, the confessions in church, in Masjid and whispers in the ears of Nandi/Ganesh, in temples are live testimonies of mental relief.

Thus, mind can make/break/elevate your mind- to any level- either to be a warrior or a magician/to be a saint.

Sun & time: Sun is a live example for value of time, Kalamu (means time) and he is considered as a visible God and he travels on seven horses, now known as VIGBYOR. Seven days for a week is an accepted tradition, though it has a sound basis in Indian astronomy. Sun gives us health (Arogya.m-Bhaskar. Prasad-am). Thus, we have entered astrology- how interferes our health?

9. Astrology

Astrology- in my opinion- is a most scientifically developed subject, wherein both Philosophers and Atheists – all-fall into one line.

The original concept of Sun rotating around the earth- is proved to be a misguided observation. From that level, man discovered that earth is spinning around the Sun. Finally, he concluded that there are at least two types of motion by earth, one bhramana (self-spin)- one day, the second around Sun (Pari-bhramana)-one year. This discussion leads to another- subject related to Sun & galaxy i.e., thus have entered into the subject astrology.

Later, the concept of earth spinning within the empty space provided by 27-star galaxies- as seen through star constellation changes observed daily. The trees begin to sprout every year after winter- from Vasanth Panchami in India and seed sowing also begins then.

The earth is now known to be spinning at @ 30 km/sec-amidst the space and takes 365 days to complete one Pari-bhramana (one rotation) around the Sun. One Rasi (is 1/12th of earth's circular path or 360^0/12). The time taken to cover that space is designated as one month and thus 12 months or @365 days make one earth's rotation (Pari-bhramana) rotation around the Sun. This is the x-axial movement of earth.

The writer of the book, "The Holy Science" – Swami Yukteswar Giri Guruji elaborated the Sun and Star movement in the Milky Way.

However, Sun is in a duet with another galaxy, which is on a y-axial movement, which is again a circular path that takes 24,000 years to make one circle. It looks like one swing up and down like a spring balance for a common observer on Z-axis.

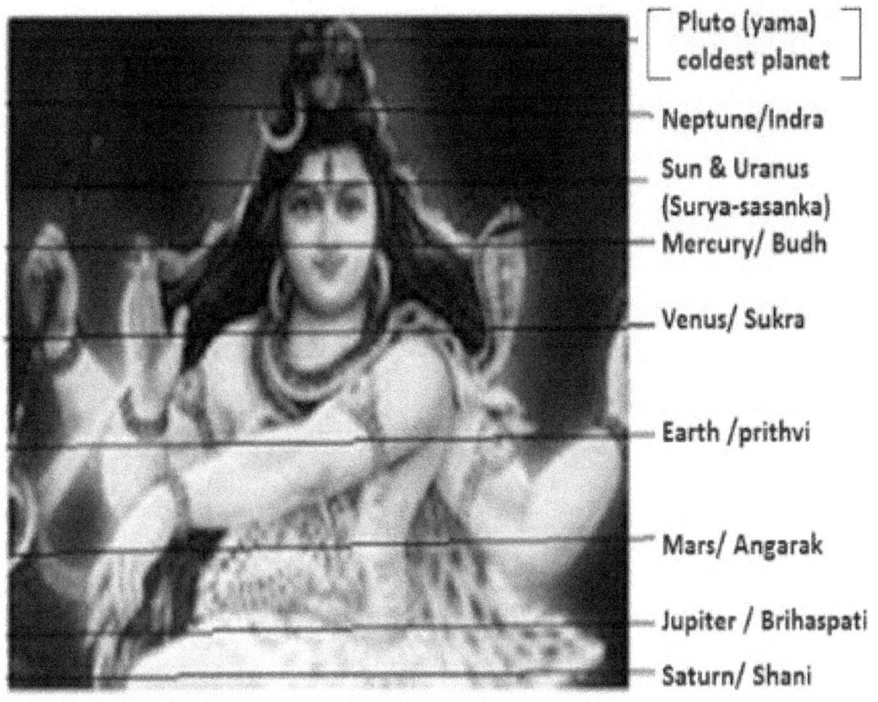

Hence, all nine graham are existing in every humanbeing and it also resembles eight chakra existing in the body- excluding Pluto

Thus, earth's movement on y-axis and on x-axis in a horizontal path,- makes- a hypothetical diagonal path for a visible observer on z-axis. When Sun comes nearer to another galaxy maximum gravity is experienced on earth. So, if this diagonal is divided into four equal parts, four yugas can be realized. Thus, each yuga needs a separate time for its movement- Krita yuga (4800), Treta yuga (3600), Dvapara yuga (2400) and Kali or (Kaali or Durga) yuga is 1200 years. See the introductory remarks by Swami Yukteswar Giri-in his book.

The third is the Sun also moving (along with many Suns) around the Centre of the Milky Way galaxy. It takes about 225 million years- known as one galactic year for one complete revolution. Sun had already completed 20 galactic years and likely to cover another 18 galactic years or more, before colliding- is the present-day prediction. But how this concept was evolved?

9.i. Observation-I: Concept of time: Kaal chakra or the concept of time is arrived by the ancient man (as elaborated by a Swamiji). It is based upon certain observations. What are they? The old houses have a concept of keeping gap for ventilation and also sunlight to enter the house,- called Manduvah which used to be an open space in the middle of the house. My grandfather used to have it in his house and later even my father-in law also had Manduvah or ventilation point in his house. Through this space Sunlight, dust and also rain can to enter into the house. The sun light travels throughout the day from one end to the other in that limited space.

It is followed by night and this pattern gets repeated every day. So, man conveniently divided that light-path of visible day time into four parts. About ¼th day time a period of just visibility in a house called tella-varu jhamu (pradosha kaal)- which begins with birds humming or crows' noise or just before sunrise. Later mid-day, afternoon, evening gets added as another jhamu each-accounting the day time. Later begins the night time, which is again divided into another four jhamu-making whole day to eight jhamu. Later, man even subdivided jhamu, how?

When one looks at someone's eye, it winks. There is a difference between a blink and a wink. One blinks with one's will, whereas wink is a natural phenomenon and the time taken for that wink is taken as vighadiya. It is further equivalent to five human respirations which is @ 24 seconds. When one counts 60 vighadiya, it becomes one Gadhiya (24 minutes) and if one counts seven and half Gadhiya it becomes one jhamu (now it is calculated to be 3hrs).

At Konark temple of Sun an understanding of the Sun's movements can be done. There are wheels for each month and time to an accuracy of two minutes can be seen. Later many Solar towers were built to know the time. Thus, Sun's shade determines time After Gadhiya & jhamu, calculations, the two-minute period is sub-divided into five vighadiya as mentioned earlier. There are erected time towers in more places in India.

In the Middle East, the count of time as fall of sand grains (Arabian culture). Greeks or Mexicans or Mongolians have kept time sense in their own way. Sand clocks, and much later, mechanical wooden clocks and finally piezo electric clocks revolutionized the time concept from month, hour, minute and even fraction of one second.

9.ii. Observation-II, Moon: The next interesting pattern is Moon changing shape every day and it repeats the pattern after @ a month. Indian Calendars are based on lunar movement. Moon takes 27 days and @8 hrs. to complete one revolution round earth.

9.iii. Survival first: If the survival of entire civilization is at stake, what to do? Swami Yukteswar Giri was being advised by his guru- Babaji to translate all vital knowledge into English language. Whenever asteroid comes, it comes at a terrible speed and gives no time for any rescue or thinking. If it collides with earth, where is the way-out? The biggest planet in Sun's galaxy, Jupiter recently experienced an asteroid, Shoemaker levy-9 strike. Jupiter survived due to its large size (1300 times the earth). If earth were to experience a similar strike, nothing on earth can survive.

What are the negative indicators in human survival now and why such confidential information was made public now?

9.iv. Negative indicators: Scientifically studies of virgin ice clusters in Antarctica suggest cooling of earth's crust occurs after every @ 10,000 years!

A. With dwindling resources, doom's day is fast coming – as depicted in another book 'The Doom's Day'?

> For example, the present consumption is @ > three million Tons of crude oil per one week in India in 1990's-which is one of the lowest in the world. This when added to the consumption of gas, coal and wood by all nations- it leads to an astronomical figure on energy consumption.

> But, when these resources petrol, coal & gas-are no longer available or not much in use, a sudden cooling of earth's crust is anticipated if petrol reserves end or- ice-age can recur!

> For example, in Telugu language- sarvari is the year 2020 and interpretation led to epidemic arrival & covid-19 struck. This forced lockdowns in India causing less petroleum consumption- which in turn resulted in surplus rainfall.

B. To make the situation worse,-what will happen to earth if an asteroid strike earth? The Hindustan Times published an article (Jan, 2002) suggesting that an asteroid twice the size of New York City is going to strike the Earth- as per old Indian astrology in the year 2212. Probably turbulence or comet collision was predicted several years back in Mexican calendar and it has no further calendar is carved on the stone-after 2010 no prediction done. Even USA was worried of the year2000 and invited many scientists into computer investigations.

Coming to the present day, what will be the fate of the present porous Earth- if it is to take a sudden impact- of the kind-Shoemaker Levi-9 that occurred upon Jupiter in this decade?- Nothing left!

C. The prediction of Yogi Veera-Brahmendra Swami in AP is corroborative to the above findings. The phenomenon like-the greenhouse effect or sea water inundating more lands or melting of Arctic and Antarctic ice.

   The virgin clusters of Antarctica revealed ice-age after every@ 10.000 years and thus another catastrophe to the entire earth or Pralaya kaal- an Indian concept-is to arrive.

D. Reduction of ozone layer around earth that caused a hole in the protective ozone layer is a real burning problem now. The world is in a crisis as less ozone layer in turn permits direct UV light penetration to earth- making scars on the human skin- a predicted phenomenon.

E. The tidal waves are set to inundate more lands of earth is a known possibility- according to the modern science. Hence, a near brink of existing civilization-is visible from all sides as written in Doom's Day book. But nuclear energy may prolong human survival later.

   So, Yukteswar Giri suggested the earth entering into Aquarius phase is also closer to the pralaya-kaal. The modern science predictions – also are looking closer to the above facts.

   Then, let us look into some more old observations.

F. If one witnesses a celestial dance in a Kuchipudi way of depiction of Shiva and Parvati, there are sudden and brisk movements by Shiva and Parvati. Further, when Parvati is nearer, majority of satellites of Shiva are on left side of Shiva (say), and Parvati – with her satellites on right side- at that time in a duet.

Here Shiva bends and passes below the arm of Parvati and vice-versa- that too-with full speed. This means the satellites of Shiva and Parvathi were cris-crossing each other then. The structure of Shiva, as shown earlier confirm Sun moves along with his satellites.

But there is a possibility of Shiva losing some satellite to Parvati or vice versa. It is where Uranus, which moves around Shiva's neck- played a vital role. During the last meeting, it is said that Uranus lost one satellite & in that process, Shiva captured it- which is said to be origin of Mars!

So, beyond doubt that Sun is in a duet with another galaxy in a fixed rhythm – on Y-axis. The month of February is the smallest in solar calendar and Shiv-ratri is also celebrated exactly on that night. So, both Solar and Lunar calendars confirm this point and is designated as lingodbhava.

G. Lingodbhava: Every year, night of Shivaratri is celebrated as lingodbhava. This is closest distance in the duet between Shiva and Parvati or the two galaxies every year, but closest occurs once in @24000 years.

The path of the rotation on Milky Way is thus the third dimension that takes one galactic year for completion of one round. Making Vada with a hole in the centre (called gari is made on the auspicious death-day puja)- is a tribute to that black hole and also thanks to our fore-fathers gave us a good hemoglobin, which is also of similar shape.

9.v: Observation – III, Sun's movement: Coming back to our naked eye observations, when one sees with a naked eye, there is a movement of Sun from Karkata Rekha to Makara Rekha in winter and vice versa in summer on the earth. In fact, in this process, earth faces the gravitational pull by Sun twice in a year needing a strong course correction @ 22nd June- the longest day (for Indians) and @ 22nd December – the shortest day (for Indians).

The impact of this axial shift is reverse to Australians. It resulted in six weather seasons in India.

9.vi: Satellites of Sun: Is that only earth is moving around the Sun. Adityaya… somaya.. Mangal-aya…. Budha-yacha. Guru…. Sukra. Sanir -Bhaschaha, raahave – ketave namaha"- is the complete sloka. When one day is deciphered into 27-star influences in 24 hours, the next day begins with the remaining graham. When the pattern was studied with nine grahams further-by keeping Sun as the first graham after seven days and this pattern is getting repeated after seven days. Thus, one week is seven days only and not nine days.

Here, Bhoomi (earth) is also being influenced by moon and moon-is the nearest of all grahams that influence humans.

If Sun and moon (Surya and Chandra) are excluded, there are only five grahams left in a week & the order is as in above sloka except Venus which has reverse impact.

They are arranged according to their neighborhood to earth. Here, rahu influence is accounted on Saturday and ketu influence is accounted on Tuesday, making 7day-a-week, calculating impact of nine in seven days. This data is based upon the star distances from the Sun as the parameter.

Adityaya	means	Sun	Sunday	aditya	Ravivaar
Soma ya	means	Moon	Monday	soma	Somvaar
Mangalaya	means	Mars	Tuesday	Mangal, kuja, angarak	Bhaumavaar
Budhayacha	means	Mercury	Wednesday	budha	Budhvaar
Guru	means	Jupiter	Thursday	deva guru	Brihaspativaar
Sukra	means	Venus	Friday	rakshas Guru	Sukravaar
Shani...r.	means	Saturn	Saturday	shani	Shanivaar

Astrology as suggested by S.V. Narayana in Eenadu newspaper dated 2nd October 2016 again once clarified that there are nine grahams including Sun- with Budh, Sukra, Bhoomi, Angarak, Brihaspati, Shani, Varun, Indra & Yama are as in below chart.

A. Budh (Mercury) is the satellite closest to Sun and also hence the hottest. It takes 58 day-15 hrs-30 min for one bhramanam (self-spin) and needs only 88 days for one paribhramanam (rotation around the Sun). It has no satellite but a scar of flowing metals due to heat and hence the old scholars thought it to be mercury. It is fourth in the sloka. Its temperatures may exceed 1500^0C and is known as business planet-Apollo by Romans.

B. Sukra, the most shining (morning star) that needs that needs 243 days-14 minutes one bhramanam (self-spin) and 225 days for one paribhramanam (rotation around the Sun). Sukra has no satellite, but rotates in opposite direction— means Sun rises in west on it or clockwise. It is also a hotter planet with temp exceeding @ 500 degrees centigrade. It is called Kavala graham or twin planet. It is also called the Goddess of love/beauty-depicts its mode of influence on humans. Sukra is also linked to semen & also to guru- Sukracharya.

C. Earth: Our Earth is the densest planet in solar system with self-spin and its bhramana kaal is one day and its paribhramana kaal is one year. It is also called the blue planet as more than 70% is water which looks blue from a distance among the Solar group of planets. It has one satellite moon which does paribhramana round the earth at a speed of 11.8 km/sec. It takes 27 days, 7 hours and 43 minutes- to make one rotation round the earth. Moon is 1/81 size of earth and its gravity is 1/6th of earth.

D. Angarak or Kuja or red planet (Angarak — means angry- the planet Mars) is considered to have been separated from Varun and has two satellites with it. It is red (aruna) graham or kuja or the god of war as Greeks call it. Mars's orbital period is 687 (Earth) days and its solar day is only slightly longer than an Earth Day and thus a Martian day looks similar. But Martian year is equal to 1.8809 Earth's year or 1 year, 320 days, and 18.2 hours.

E. Guru (Brihaspati) or Jupiter is the largest planet serving as satellite around the Sun. It is the largest graham of Sun & nearly 1300 times the size of earth and has fastest spin of 9hrs-50 min-30 seconds for one bhramana kaal (self-spin). It needs 12 years for one rotation (its paribhramana kaal) around Sun with 18 major satellites and is said to have @67 satellites in toto. protecting the Sun's galaxy.

It means that before earth makes one day, Jupiter completes more than two rounds bhramana and about to complete the third. Hence it can shake earth's weather pattern through gravitational pull, making draught or surplus water. In size and spin-Guru is far ahead of Mars or (in other words, the Indian story – Ganesh won and Kartikeya lost – is linked for easy memory. Further after losing Kartikeya became red faced-depicting the color of Mars).

Here, Agarak or Mars- makes one day in its spin in nearly 29 hours and that time is enough to Guru or Brihaspati or Jupiter (huge size Ganesh),-to spin thrice for one spin of Mars. But Jupiter is nearly 1300 times size of earth, while Mars is smaller than earth. Hence, the Boss or Sun (or Lord Shiva) finds that the planet Guru is superior to the red planet.

Corollary: Boss blesses that person, who visits him often!

F. Shani (Saturn) is the satellite with bhramana-kaal self-spin) 10 hrs. 14 min. that takes 30 years to make a single rotation around Sun and has maximum number satellites nearly 24 of good size. The second largest planet in solar family is Shani and has sp.gr around 0.69. It also holds @62 satellites all put in toto.

It means Shani's spin and speed is just behind that of Jupiter (guru). But due to long distance, Shani needs thirty years one rotation around Sun (paribhramana). It is also called as cruel planet or golden planet. But it is said that Shani by itself can not cause any negative effect. It is our dark deeds, that come to light through this planet.

Corollary: Only victor is noticed, but not the second.

G. Varun (Uranus): Uranus is the seventh planet for the Sun.

The Uranus's orbit has a unique configuration and widely differ from the other planets. Uranus travels in Sun's rotational axis and thus it runs parallel to Sun with a unique path – with bhramana is 17 hours, 14 minutes and paribhramana is 84 years. g. Varun (Uranus): Uranus is the seventh planet for the

Sun. The Uranus's orbit has a unique configuration and widely differ from the other planets. Uranus travels in Sun's

Name	Diameter in kms.	Distance from Sun in kms.	Direction of spin	One rotation w.r.to Sun
Sun	1,390,000	0	0	0
Mercury	4.878	57,910,000	clockwise 58 day -15 hrs-30 min self spin	88 days
Venus	12,104	108,200,000	Anti-clockwise 243 days-14 min.	225 days
Earth	12,756	149,600,000	clockwise one day	one year- 1 satellite
Mars	6,794	227, 940,000	clockwise 24 hours, 39 min	1.9 years, 2 satellites
Jupiter	142,984	778,330,000	clockwise fastest spin of 9hrs-50 min-30 sec	12 years, 18 satellites
Saturn	120,536	1,329,400,000	clockwise spin 10 hrs 14 min.	30 years 24 satellites
Uranus	51,118	2,870,990,000	clockwise	84 years, 5 satellites
Neptune	49.528	4,504,300,000	Anti-clockwise	168 years
Pluto	2,340	5,913,520,000	clockwise	248 years

Uranus has large amounts of methane gas is said to be on it and hence called green planet or Varun or God in the sky. (It is rotational axis and thus it runs parallel to Sun with a unique path-with bhramana is 17 hours,   14 minutes and paribhramana is 84 years known as Kunti of Mahabharata, because it has five moons namely Ariel, Umbriel, Miranda, Titania and Oberon. It has lost Mars, (la Kunti lost Karna in Mahabharat- is the story). Uranus is the third biggest satellite around Sun after Brihaspati and Shani in size. In fact, the new element uranium got its name after the discovery of the planet Uranus.

H. Indra (Neptune): It is a distant and one of the chilliest planets that rotates quite opposite to earth's direction. Indra (Neptune) that takes 18 hrs.' and 26-minute bhramana and its paribhramana is 165 years. It is depicted as half-moon on the head of Shiva-picture in back pages & has satellites around 14 and most important are Triton and Nerida. It takes 83 years with Sun and chooses another unknown path for 82 years.

I. Yama (Pluto): It is the chilliest planet and most of the scientists when met is Czechoslovakia in 2002 considered it-not to be in our solar system, but its presence recorded in traditional sloka as Yama- means – death nearby.

Hence Sun has only six satellites and the rest been closely moving nearer to Sun's galaxy. Here, Varun moves parallel around the Sun. The mantra suggests as 'Surya- sasanka- vahni- nayanam', where one eye is Sun and another eye is the green planet Uranus. Here, Shiva is considered as Sadashiv (ever existing) with all stars as concentric rings, making his body. (as in first page of astrology) Further, all eight chakras exist in every human. Here, Pluto is said to cause serious mental disturbances.

The Sky is- the fifth of the panca-mahabhoot that control our health. In simple words, the humans are considered as simple expressions of the Navagraha influences upon earth.

These influences are concentric rings from the head of Shiva (Sun), up to Saturn as shown above in Lord Shiva structure, which exist in every human. So, he comes under the influences of Ravi, Budh- Sukra-Bhumi – Kuja – Guru – Shani-Rahu and Ketu in a serial order!

How it is connected to our health chakra or how it is co-related with diseases- is given in ayurvedic theory. These grahams are placed in eight places around the Sun and worshipped as Navagraha, where the priest is fully conscious of their place (See – in Satyanarayana-vratam puja). If one observes the Navagraha placements in any temple, the faces of all satellites are in different directions. How this concept was arrived at?

It is an observation of several generations & needs calculations. Now, the earth takes one day or 24 hrs. or to be exact- 23hrs, 56 min. 4.091 seconds to make one bhramana kaal (one day). Similarly moon takes @27 days, 7hrs, 43 minutes and 12 seconds for one pari-bhramana around the earth are NASA-USA calculations.

9.vii. Observation-IV, Star galaxies: The earth, during its one-day spin, it crosses all 27-star galaxies in one-day circular spin. Starting from the star Ashwini up-to Revathi & all are depicted as below:

1. Ashwini: This is made of three stars that mimic the face of the horse, visible in the star's constellation.

2. Bharani too, there will be three stars that depict a distant triangle- but with stretched length.

3. Kritika: There are six stars like a curve like 2nd day moon or like a communist symbol or kodavali or like dhatri (the grass cutter knife- commonly used).

4.   Rohini: This star galaxy is like a Tonga or a cart.

5.   Mrigasira: These stars as trio depict like an animal head.

6.   Arudra: Here the galaxy looks like a pogadam.

7.   Punarvasu: There is a combination of five stars that look like a bow (Dhanush).

8.   Pushyami: This is group just similar with minor changes from above.

9.   Alesha: There are seven stars in hap-hazard fashion.

10. Magha (Makah): It looks like a palanquin made of eight stars.

11. &12. Pubba & Uttara: This is a group made of two pairs of stars looks like a square, before crossover to another group.

12. Hasta: There are five stars in a group like an elephant's tusk.

13. Chitra or Chita: It is a single star like a pearl. 25 & 26. Poorva Bhadra & Uttara Bhadra: Again, two pairs of stars in the galaxy.

14. Swati: It is again a bright Manickam shaped star.

15. Visakha (Sarika): This is a star galaxy in a wheel shaped order.

16. &18. Anuradha & Jyeshta: This group is made of six stars like an umbrella and is covered as two stars- Anuradha and Jyeshta.

17. Moola: When there are five stars that look like a vessel.

18. &21. Poorvashada & Uttarashada: Both stars close by as a double.

19. Sravanam: There are three stars that look like a flute, means one line.

20. Dannisha: There will be five stars that look like a maddela (tabla).

21. Satabhisham: It is made of hundreds of stars in a line. That means it can be the opening into many galaxies in the Universe.

22. Revathi: The stars in the galaxy resemble like a fish with 32 stars.

Thus, in nutshell, a huge universe around the earth- is conveniently divided into 27-star galaxies. Now, next question arises such as- how many satellites exist in Sun's galaxy? Thus, the next aspect of astrology, is a big subject-with the cosmic constellations around Sun.

There are many Suns on the path of Milky Way. In Indian concept-every star in the galaxy is treated as God or devta or graham or devta Swaroopa.

9.viii: Stars exert influence:- Here, when one looks into the sky from earth, many stars are located. In physics there is a parameter called G, which determines the attraction between two objects-depending upon their mass, distance and speed. All distances and the position of Sun vis-a vis other satellites already given, but can be visualized horizontally.

The above structure of grahams (satellites of Sun)-that are laid in order as horizontal or X-axis as below. If this set seen vertical or Y-axis-the meditative posture of Shiva as given earlier visualized.

Then, it is like a triangle or a bell, wherein satellites starting from mercury up to Saturn make a wide base with Sun as the pivot-with Saturn – being at the lowest at the base.

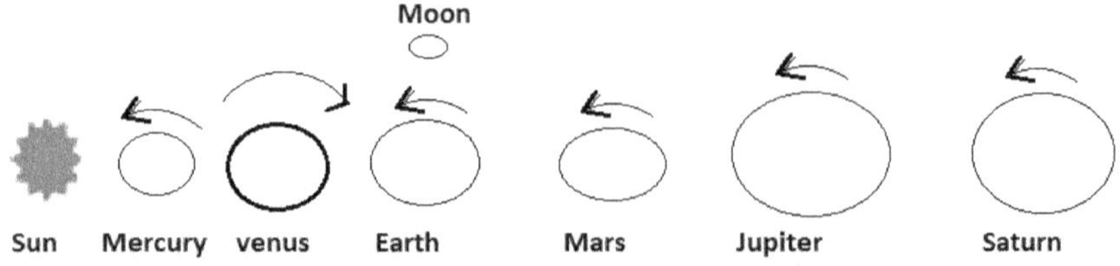

The ayurvedic-asta chakra also match to the exact eight satellite positions around Sun & depicted as Shiva above.

So, Shiva (Sun) and its satellites are spinning like a bell. It means as satellite is away from the Sun, the spinning axis of that satellite expands as gravity falls. But, Shiva's swing with Parvathi is upward and down-ward or vertical movement is the closest on Shiv-ratri, which is accounted as the Lingodbhava time. This gives an excellent understandable picture of the spatial movement of Sun and its satellites.

9.ix: Pious number: How the pious number 108 had arisen? If the area of entire sky used by our earth for making a huge circle in space- is divided into 12 fractions, making each part is of 30^0, (Rasi). Thus, 12 Rasi (30^0x 12 =360^0) makes one revolution by earth around the Sun, or one year. But this movement is within 27 groups of stars. Their- LCM, it means – of both 27 & 12, makes 108. Since Sun moves along with satellites, the shape of Shiva-made-up of nine stars also with gravitational pressures of push and pull- during the entire length of movement. Thus, there are 108 variations or Shiva has 108 loka. According to Swami Yukteswar Giri, in the year 2499, the earth is going to enter Leo/Aquarius phase.

9.x: Pancangam (observation V): Based on the date, time, and place of birth (longitude and latitude), a person's health/disease, winner/looser, wealth/poverty is predicted. Then, how to overcome the impact?- Coming to the nine grahams of Sun, one will be tempted to know which aspects are present in pancangam (Indian calendar), called pancangam- has five variables- namely, tithi (moon movement), vaaram (the satellite as graham to remember every day), and nakshatram, which are common to all humans on earth. Based upon their date, place and time of birth, two more factors, yogam and karanam gets added. These are specific to a particular area and particular person. Based upon such data the predictions are made.

9.xi: Sun-& seasonal diseases: Sun during its rotation enters makara rasi- beginning Uttar Ayan and in the same way Sun enters Karkataka rasi beginning Dakshin Ayan in India- that brings in the seasonal diseases. They are a, b, c, d, e & f as below:

A. Vasanth ritu- (Chaitra-Vaisakha @Mar- Apr) – it is with kapha Prokop (outburst); Here ritu means seasonal weather.

B. Grisham ritu- (Jyeshta-Asada- @May-June), it is with vata sanchaya (packaged) & with kapha.

C. Varsha ritu- (Sravan-Bhadrapada- @Jul- Aug), it is with pitta packaged & vata active.

D. Sharad ritu- (Aswiyuja-kartika-@Sept-Oct), it is with pitta outburst & vata also there.

   e.Hemanta ritu- (Margasira- Pushya- @Nov-Dec), it is associated with pitta (indigestion).

E. Sisira ritu- (Magha-Phalguna- @Jan-Feb), it is with kapha sanchaya-(packaged). Thus, every season brings disturbances in our health. So, one adopts the path of appeasement.

9.xii. Appeasement of stars: In case of bad days, astrology gives some indications wherein pacifications can make a difference.

This is done by some colored stones, grains and even metal pieces, colors or colored clothes are used for appeasement of any selected graham.

These nine grahams have each one cereal grain. Not only grain, one precious stone, one suitable colored cloth, one medicinal herb each, and finally have their own shape. The sufferer is thus advised to worship the troubling graham, by offering clothes, cereals, even distribute cooked food and proceed further by forgetting the losses. It boosts the morale of the person and provides proper mindset for survival. Here, the Yogam (is there any possibility of gain or loss in your horoscope.

This yogam is of 27 variations; Karanam is the parting star's impact and is of eleven variations. The astrologers are the best judges for the discussion.

9.xiii: Herbs and pacification: Here there lies the last aspect- that the nine grahams are also being linked to medicinal herbs for havan (sacred fire). It is here astrology is linked to our health and herbs are suggested to be put into havan or grow the herb or water the herb for appeasement of that graham. Thus, there are 27 herbs for 27 stars & in doing so, the person's vision sharpens!

Hence, Astrology fore warns about up- coming crisis in advance. If one looks to the events philosophically, by sitting idle and let stars to act, he will die of hunger and starvation.

9.xiv: Overcome the dilemma: Lord Buddha had a dilemma-after self-realization- as he preferred starvation. Then, a tribal woman gave goat's milk and forced recovery Buddha. When he became conscious, she questioned him "Even if you realize truth Sir, how can you talk about your achievements to others or guide them without being alive? So, Sir I request you to please be alive and teach others of your findings!" Then he began to preach the path of peace by shunning all violence.

Day	Planet	Colour	Gem	grain	Metal
sunday	ravi	Red	Ruby/ kempu	Wheat	Bronze
mon	chandra	White	Pearl/mutyam	Paddy/ rice	Lead
tue	Mangal /kuja	Red	Coral/pogadam	Red lentil	copper
tue	Ketu	Multi colour	Cat's eye/ vydhuryam/lapislazuli	Horse gram	Red stone
Wed	budh	Green	Emerald/paccha	Green gram	mercury
Thurs	guru	Yellow	Yellow sapphire /pushyaragam	Yellow split pea, Chana dal	gold
Fri	sukra	White	Diamond/vajram	Soya gram	silver
Sat	shani	Blue	Blue sapphire /neelam	Sesame	Iron and steel
Sat	Rahu	Black	gomedhicam/ Zircon/sardonya	Black gram	Black stone

Religion is a path from darkness to light. Sankara-acharya is followed by Ramanuja-acharya, Madhava-acharya, Jesus Christ and Prophet Mohammed. The recent Avtar, Adi Shankara consolidated Vedic rules and travelled throughout India-when no transport and no electricity available. Then, he suggested to make fire using wood friction methods, which is a practice even today for doing hawan or sacred fire.

He never used motor vehicle during his all-India travel.

Thus, we come to the end of astrology with many unknown factors affecting in astrology. They can be understood only through a scholar. This, thus completes all invisibles.

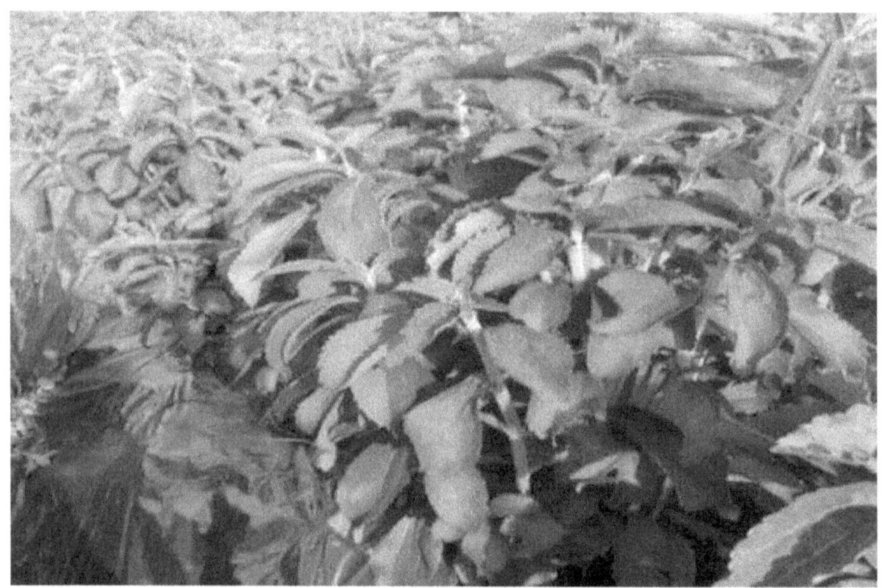

Ajwain-ka-patta, consumable

10. Summary & Conclusions

A sincere attempt has been made to look into all important factors affecting a normal health. As a natural product scientist & drug analyst with touch in herbal medicine, I only looked into the basic facts. Thus, I am neither an ayurveda scholar nor a physician, nor a botanist nor an astrologer to deal with these subjects nor I can predict the future.

Once upon a time nearly forty years back, with my liver was partly damaged, plus doctors warned me of risk of heart attack. In later years, I had already faced two modern surgeries. It is beyond doubt that such treatments were impossible in the age-old system. I am indebted to the modern drugs and no doubt, these are good. But the physician now, depends upon modern detection techniques that add to the cost of treatment!

The old days of detection of trouble is through observation of simple pulse like- late Dolma of Sino-Tibetan medicine no longer exist now. People forgot that medicine is a stimulus for recovery, but only the body has to act in cure.

Some medicines can be toxic affecting the digestive organs, including liver & kidney. Overcoming their negative impact- is by adding more medicines. It is a vicious circle wherein no outlet is possible.

In case of ayurveda, only natural products are used as medicines, though some treatments as vati/tablet. The chances their being less digested is rare. There are many toxic medicines even in ayurveda too. These negative effects are recorded as vipaka. Hence, a physician's advice with herb consumption & follow up is essential.

The vital point to remember is that even when no industrial development, ayurveda existed and even now it is existing- with its name not mentioned.

Once it so-happened that I and my doctor were on a dinner party. The doctor was staring at my plate. The next day, I visited him for a routine check-up. That physician commented that any medicine is useless for you as you lack control over eating food. So, eat food for living, but not to live for eating food!

Upon his advice, I started adding mode salads to my diet and tried to reduce salt in diet. After reading the literature, I find that there is a direct relation-ship between the salt consumed and the hunger.

It means less salt will ultimately result in less hunger as hydrochloric acid needs salt break-up in stomach to generate it. Next, it is excess tea with sugar that generates more acid with gastric trouble.

After my retirement, when the health problems cropped up again- the doctor suggested me to reduce meat consumption and added more medicines.

Then, I decided to come out of modern drugs and its tests as far as possible. I started to look into the old way of living of the people-between Himalayas and Indian ocean- is named as Sanatana dharma and it has inbuilt controls on health- that is ayurveda. This Indian way of living, is our religion, Hinduism!

Ultimately, I recognized three enemies of the body, namely, salt, carbohydrates, foods of animal origin & finally oil rich food add lethargy too. The old Indian way is that- where no work-no food.

Lord Shiva is known to have practiced upon long fast and who wants to see him also need to fast. Fasting is a method of appeasement.

Another way is that in ayurveda fresh water collected is reduced to 1/4th level, cooled and filtered. Why so? Scientifically such water becomes rich in magnesium and these ions enter every cell to reduce the sodium content-an astonishing technique!

Your blood pressure is nothing but a sodium/potassium ratio. Drinking magnesium rich water so prepared above will reduce salt elimination. I used to see red sandal dolls-lying in the puja room in the old days.

"In my opinion, vegetarianism is a luxury-possible only when-one eliminates excess animals. Thus, meat lovers are an asset to the society."

I started growing essential herbs needed for health. I preferred kalmegh as it can be grown at home & is present in more than twenty liver extracts with capacity to cure even jaundice & digestive disorders. This basic herb for survival- was brought from Srisailam, AP. I also presented herbs as photos in the text.

Then, I changed regular diet with salads and began morning walk. In about three years, my body swung to recovery-that too with minimal medicines.

Coming back into the subject, I started analyzing each procedure starting from hydrotherapy, faith therapy, food therapy, Ganesh puja therapy and also spice therapy. They form part-I of health. Next part-II therapies with many herbs, though the details are suggestive in nature, consultation of physician essential. The next is to look into all invisible parameters that impact our health-accounted as part-III health.

A person is in water- at least half bust level. Then reverse osmosis begins in full swing into the kidneys. The time spent is regulated by the priest chanting the mantra 108 times or @½ hr. Modern day swimming in river or swimming pool- also extends a similar benefit, provided no chemical is added into the pond waters.

Another is cow urine and cow dung use explained already in subject preview. It eliminates even some hard-core diseases struck in your body. Ganesh puja-offers several lessons, including choosing a right time for plant collection & important herbs.

In India, prolonged use of vegetables to cure human system- as practiced- since ages as in home therapy. Hence, naturopathy is embedded in the Indian way of living. This is followed by rearing animals, for milk and meat, which keeps eco-balance in nature. Even snakes and scorpion festivals exist every year.

The ayurvedic theory, mind and astrology have multiple impacts on our body. The soul comes to life with a list of desires, which get vibrated to mind and accepted or rejected by the intellect (brain)- based upon their practicality.

Finally, all acts follow a path of karma. "Buddhi- karma- anusarini". Path of karma is a superstition, one may call-but is a reality. Karma is an individual dilemma. But the soul is the driver of the body.

If one goes through Garuda Puranam, the mechanism to free, a dead person's soul – is well explained. If the mind is properly directed, the person can be a magician or can be a great Saint.

Adi-Shankara, who came like a bubble to teach several Vedic rules. Later came many Saints. Shirdi Sai baba and Satya Sai Baba suggested to lead life without worries. I had an opportunity to see Satya-Sai-Baba of Puttaparthi and heard his discourses.

The real picture of God is presented by Bhagavan Satya Sai Baba as a lamp (from darkness to light) and presented all religions around it- meaning a religious path is towards the lamp. so, God is nir-akara, shapeless or ananta or unlimited.

Sun- a big hydrogen bomb-ever exploding- providing light and energy for our survival-& a true God. Thus, there are all- path breakers – fitting in to the saying 'daivam. Manasa-roupena'. God comes in a human form is the meaning and it is also the exact saying of Lord Krishna in Bhagavat Gita.

Astrology is the final subject that comes with four Yugas, guided by four path finders- Shiva (Krita-Yuga), Rama (Treta Yuga), Krishna (Dvapara Yuga) & Durga (Kali or Kaali Yuga) – this yuga division is in Vedic- astrology. If the God is shapeless why so many Gods in each Yuga?

Gayatri mantra is said to have been developed by Seer-s to activate the beads of the spinal cord. Lord Shiva suggested- work is worship. He used ox as vehicle and plough fields with cereals for production of food grains.

The next is- hold money and comfort or money- based path-reaching goal with satisfaction Vishnu (Jai Rama-krishna-govinda-Narayana) and the final the knowledge-based path- leading towards zero or nirguna tatwa. Thus, three stalwarts for each path exists- Brahma (creator, truthful vision), Vishnu (propagator, money holding), or Shiva (power) exist.

Here, loss or gain of power is like- two shades of a moon. There is another angle to moon is like Indra. The loss or gain of power is compared to Neptune. Thus, Neptune has a unique path of 164 years- with half the time in Sun's orbit and half the time in another invisible path. This is exact representation of change of power- on earth. For example, when Neptune left Sun's path in 1999 and exactly that year-king Mahindra lost power & was killed! When Julius Caesar was about to be killed, he was being fore-warned of his murder, he did not respond to warnings. Thus, all Astro-predictions are powerful.

Then, one may ask a question such as how to elevate ourselves. Adi-Shankara had preached say Govind-a and adds further as below;

"Sat-sangatve. Nissangatva". From a good company to no company;--." nis-sangatve nir-mohatwa"... from that a clean mind with no desires;- "nirmohatve. Nischalatatwa".- then one reaches a steady state;-- "nischal-tatwe. Jeevan muktihi"...-reach a state free from rebirth!

In the next, like a saint be jubilant to say "Jai- sat- chit-Ananda"- means 'wo.h victorious soul',- with physical and mental happiness and reach a state free from rebirth.

Thus, all these methods are to elevate people mentally and reach salvation at the earliest. This ends our total discussion on health. The saints/sanyasi stopped doing wrong deeds to elevate them. Thus, good deeds come to elevating mind and soul becomes lighter and free! Thus, Buddhism, Jainism, Christianity & even Islam were evolved for better living and one who guides people to a correct path can be designated as a prophet/God.

Modern medicines: Thescientists- while doing electron mapping of morphine, found that its pattern matches with anal-gin in one dimension- this led to discover more analgesics through synthetic means. Similarly, Keir's triangle for diabetic drugs mattered wherein many sugar substitutes were discovered.

Here, chemistry not only- clarified the chemical content in the herbs but also helped in locating their effective groups. The Nobel Prize in chemistry (2018) had gone to the group, who managed production of enzymes, chemicals and proteins by modifying the genes of bacilli in a test tube.

This led to production large number of biochemical- all thanks to the petro- revolution. But what will happen when petrol production ceases?

The human cells have a pore size less than of potassium ion. Hence, only very few elements in the periodic table have a direct impact by entering human cell pores. Potassium is captive ion inside the cell while sodium freely goes in and out.

This osmotic play of control for blood pressure work through sodium excretion-which bath in rivers and ponds do. If any metal ion beyond the size of potassium if taken internally, it either breaks human cell or any other cell or act like a scavenger in eliminating several unusual bacilli cells- including cancer cells and this is what Shilajit or konda-malam-is known to do. I have used rasarath a patanjali mercury- complex- three sacks guided by ayurvedic physician to eliminate initial growth of suspected cancer cells.

How to go back to nature:

I remembered my breakfast of childhood, it was tarwani (rice boiled hot water put into a pot with salt added to it). Tarwani is slowly fermented, with every day addition of cooked & leftover rice in the night into it, acting as a a natural refrigerator. If child drinks a glassful in the morning, he will never face sun-stroke.

Plus, achar and rice in tarwani is a good breakfast too. Further the boiled and filtered rice is an asset with less starch and good for the elders as soluble starch is reduced. This fluid is stable for months. But once in a year the pot is replaced with new- an age-old refrigerator for cooked rice!

Another preservative is pickling. A cut raw mango pieces, of width @2-3 cm x length 8-12 cm – are collected and cleaned with dry muslin. Such cut-mango pieces fresh (@3kg), mixed with raw mustard powder (½ kg), red chili powder (1/2 kg), and salt (@850 gms)- preferably low sodium – rock salt, with methre (trigonella – feonum-glaucum) seeds @50 gm. and oil @ one liter- stored in a porcelain jar for years. This pickle called avakaya, supplies mango for years that too with vitamin – C. It is age-old practice since ages.

In conclusion, unless you practice, how can you tell someone about survival methods? Once, Guru Drona said 'always speak truth' – all students uttered so, but Yudhishthira did not speak (Mahabharata)- when questioned by his guru, he said,-Sir I will practice now onwards!

According to my elders (predecessors), I have to improve my daily routine (dina-charya). So first and foremost, point is to mend the body to habituate a regular rhythm. I remembered the Prime Minister Morarji Desai. His regular walking exercise benefited him at the age of @80 years. So, I changed my working time table and began morning walk that has brought many friends (more than twenty) with healthy discussions on philosophy and gossip & jokes extra.

For example, taking water before walk- is an acupressure as it sends water & magnesium into the body with quick walk- to displace other obstructive organic/inorganic ions in the supply lines (no medicine used here). I am better than what I was – with lesser medicines on about three years.

Plus, one can locate plants by the names. Ippa tree- dead is worshipped as Srimukhalinga, Sirimanu festival is using imli tree & place called chintala valasa exist. At,Vibhitaki tree, Karaka-chettu polamamba exists and white Calotropis procera becomes sweta-rka Ganesh in Khazipet and a gaint nim tree is cut every twelve years to make Lord Jagannath.

Similarly, mangadu means mango forest in Tamil Nādu and it is also known as chuta vanam. It is where tapo Kamakshi temple was built. Ficus religiosa or Aegle marmelos are worshipped in the name of Lord Shiva and Badari tree gives the name to Lord Badrinath or Vishnu.

Thus, amudala valasa means castor tree rich place!

My parents used to force us to wash hands legs and face just outside the house, with bucket-full of water before entering the house, in outer verandah (gallery). Some saints used masks for mouth & nose long back. My (late) grandfather, after market visit- used to take a regular bath by dipping all clothes into water.

Now modern houses are made with rooms next to the main road and windows into stretching even to neighbor's house & no space for gallery. What happens if small pox or chicken pox or covid-19 strikes in the neighborhood?

Thus, my aim is to condense available methods related to health into a single book in a simple way so that the family members who lost roots, can recover. Thanks to all readers.-P. G. Rao

My Reading References

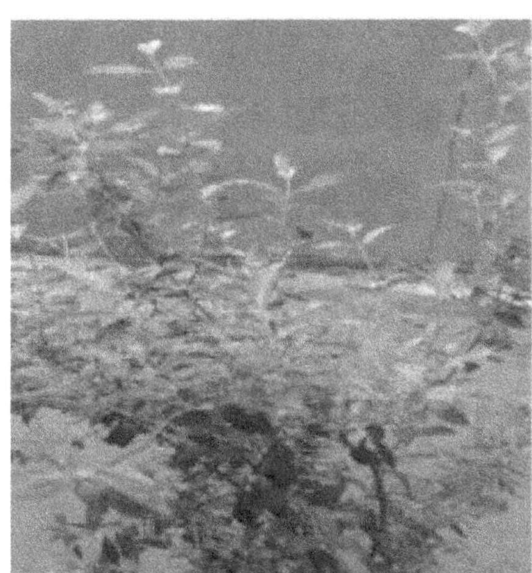

Mehandi

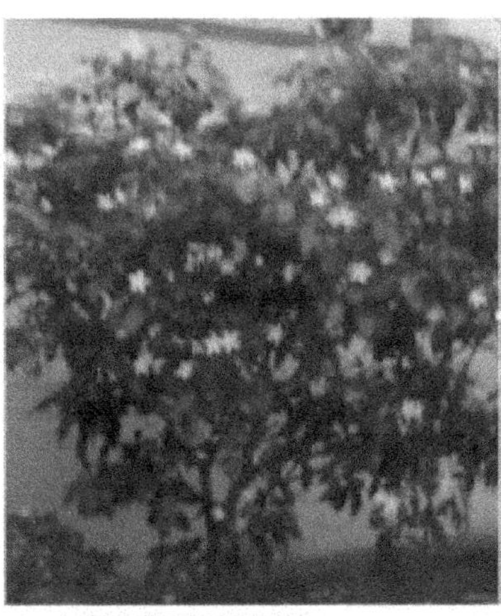

Nandi-vardhanam

1. Basic concept of disease with special reference to ayurveda and yoga; Dev Prasad Sahu; J. Res. Ay. Sid., 1981, II,376-400.

2. A second prize-Shri Hari-Om-trust-award gold medal-receipient from The Gujarat Ayurvedic University, Jamnagar, 1984.

3. Scientific evidence on the role of Ayurvedic herbal on bioavailability of drugs; C.K. Atal, Usha Zutshi, and P.G.Rao; J.Ethanopharmacol, 1981, 4, 229-232;

4. Discourses of scholars on God, Yoga, and health.

5. Herbal medicine – a modern approach- from Herbal research institute, Golconda, 1996.

6. Equilibrium studies of ternary chelates of some divalent metal ions with cephalosporins and alanine; Parushottam B. Chakrawarti, J.Ind. chem. Soc, 2000, 77, 212-219.

7. Charak samhita (English) by Sh. Bhagavan Dash, 1941

8. CSIR-R&D highlights, Risorcine-a novel CSIR drug curtails TB – treatment, Dr.P. Cheena chawla; CSIR News, March 2010, p52.

9. Ethnomedicinal and Ethno-veterinary Plants, by   M   . Venkat Ramana, Ethnobot. Leaflets, 12, 2008, 391-400.

10. The autobiography of a yogi- by Swmi Yogananda (YSS-Publications).

11. The holy science, book by Swami Yukteswar Giri. (YSS-Publications).

12. 12. The Doom's Day – book (IIIM, library)

13. Handbook of ayurvedic medicinal plants by L.D. Kapoor 1990

14. Plants as liver protectors; A. Subramaniam and P. Pushpangadan; Indian J. Pharmacol.1999, 31, 166-

15. Antioxidant and antibacterial investigations on essential oils & acetone extracts of some spices; Gurdip Singh et.al, Natural product radiance, 2009, 6(2), 114-121.

16. A series of articles by professor Ramachandran on living with diabetes in Indian Express 1993;

17. Also living with diabetes weekly series by Dr. Agarwal of diabetes forum-series-in the same paper later.

18. A handbook of notes – prepared by P. suryanarayana, 1933 (birakayala appanna pantulu dictates@1910).

19. Hand book of domestic medicine & common ayurvedic remedies by P.N.V. Kurup (ICMR), book 1978.

20. Simple remedies take a backseat, by P.G. Rao, The Hindu, April, 27, 2014,

21. More advises from friends, colleagues, relations and also elders.

22. Adsorption-desorption of heavy metal ions 2014 by S.P. Misra, a review article, Curr. Sci., 102, (4), p601-612. More from World Wide Web, with special mention to google;

Important Word Meaning - (as Understood by Me)

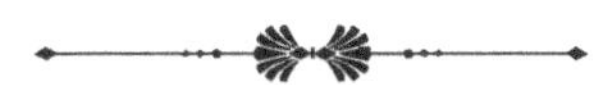

Adi Shankara – first Sankaracharya Amada – Telugu name for Yojanam Anindya – unaccused

Anna – 1/16th of an old rupee Aquarius – Zodiac orbit Ayyappa – God

Beda – 1/8th of old rupee Betha – Four finger width or @3" Bhavani – Durga

Budhi – Intelligence Charak – A sage, physician Chikitsa – remedy Chit – mind

Dabbu – a copper coin, 1/3 anna Gajam – 36 inches, one step of elephant, in my opinion Ganesh – Son of Goddess Parvati Godi in telugu – @ 4" (@width of brick/width of horse's paw) Hanuman – who served Rama Hasta, – Hand fingers laid flat Havan or Yagna or hawan- sacred ritual performed through fire Jaana – Length of one brick @9" Kani – 1/4th of anna

Kosu – Probably half a mile

Krishna – God of Dvapara – yuga

Kunta – area of irrigable land – using a well

Mahabharat – the epic

Mahatma Gandhi – Father of Indian nation

Muura – one elbow or @18" length

Paisa – 1/12th of an anna

Panca-mahabhoot – earth, water, fire, air & sky;

Parvathi – wife of Shiva Patram – leaf Puja – worship

Rama – God of Treta-yuga Samhita – compilation Sanyas renunciation, Ser – Volume @ 700ml Shanmukh – son of Shiva Shiva- God of Krita-yuga

Shivaji – a king who fought Aurangzeb Shoemaker Levi-9 – asteroid--that fell on Jupiter

Siddhi – acquired mythical powers Sushruta, – physician of@ 600 BC Swamiji – Seer or Rishi or Saint Veera-brahmendra Swami – a – revered saint in AP Viswanayaka – world leader Vyasa – author of Mahabharat Yogananda – author/autobiography of a yogi.

Yojanam – Sanskrit measure of distance

Yukteswar Giri – Revered saint

One of My Morning Walkers Group Below

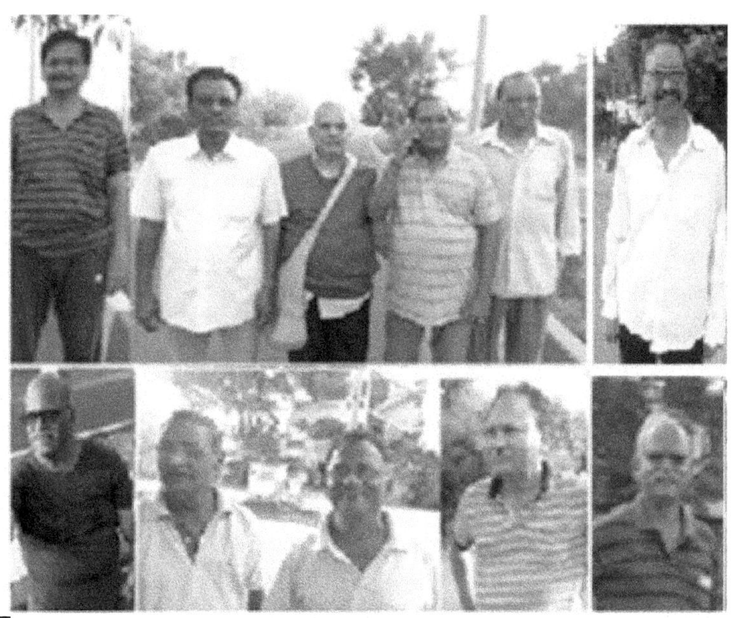

About the Author

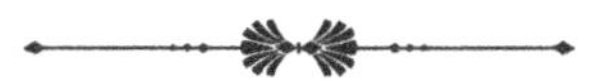

The author is a superannuated scientist of organic chemistry & worked in Natural products division, Indian Institute of Integrative Medicine (formerly Regional Research Laboratory) canal road, Jammutawi, with several publications and presentations; Made part contributions in books; A Radio-Isotopic labeling and RIA developer cum analyst; A DAAD, Scholarship holder-Germany-1980-81; Hari- om – trust awardee- a second prize- Gold medalist, 1984 (from Gujarat Ayurvedic University, Jamnagar); A member of Yogoda Satsang Society, Ranchi, 1986-89; member, Sri Bhagawan Satya Sai Seva samithi, 1986-89 & served as Secretary for Sai samithi in J&K, one year; Secretary RRL Scientific Workers Association, Jammu for one year-1991; Diploma in Herbal medicine from HRI Golconda 1995-97; Member Dhanwantari Foundation International 2011; Member of Subhasya vipra sangham, 2012.